# Pediatric Meds Made Easy

Callie Parker

Copyright © 2025 by Callie Parker

All rights reserved.

No portion of this book may be reproduced in any form without written permission from the publisher or author, except as permitted by U.S. copyright law.

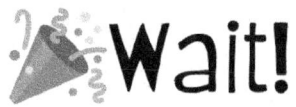 # Wait!

### Before You Dive In... Grab Your FREE Nursing Study Survival Kit!

Nursing school is no joke—that's why MadeEasy.Academy is committed to sending the ladder back down and rescuing those of you in the trenches!

Ready to study smarter, not harder? We've got exactly what you need.

Your FREE NCLEX in My Sleep Bundle Includes:

✅ Who's Dying First? The Prioritization Playbook: Because patient safety is kind of a big deal. 😅
✅ Flashcard Frenzy: Memorize or Die Trying: Pre-made Anki cards to save your sanity.
✅ WTF Does This Lab Value Mean? Cheat Sheet: No more second-guessing normal vs. "oh sh*t" levels.
✅ NCLEX Mnemonics That Stick (Like Tape on an IV Line): Memory hacks you'll actually remember.
✅ Med Math Without the Mental Breakdown: Because no one wants to commit a dosage error. 😬

 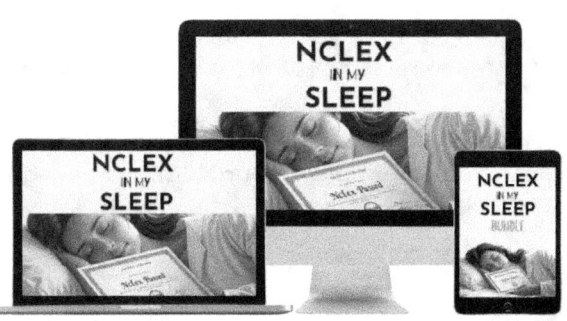

Head over to MadeEasy.Academy to grab your bundle. Let's turn nursing school stress into success!

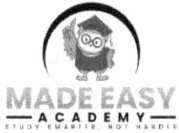

## But that's not all...

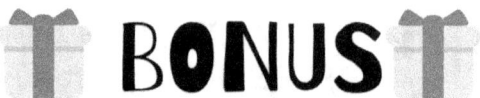

## Your Bundle Includes an Exclusive 50% OFF Discount Code for your next course at Made Easy Academy
(Launching June 1!)

At MadeEasy.Academy we don't just simplify nursing—we transform it into an effortless, memorable study process.

For each topic, you'll follow our step by step success guide:

 Step 1. Grab your cheat sheet: All key points, zero fluff.

 Step 2. Read your mnemonic poem: Clever rhymes to make information stick.

 Step 3. Take your fill-in-the-blank quiz: Test your recall without the overwhelm.

 Step 4. Complete your NCLEX challenge: Realistic practice questions with clear rationales.

 **Step 5. Walk Into the NCLEX Like a Boss:** Confident, prepared, and ready to pass.

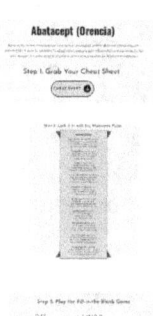
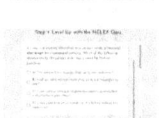
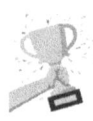

Right now, we're laser-focused on Pharmacology, but we'll soon expand into other crucial nursing topics! Have a topic you want us to cover next? Shoot us an email at hello@madeeasy.academy—we've got you!

# Contents

1. Acetaminophen (Tylenol) — 5
2. Ciprofloxacin Ophthalmic (Ciloxan) — 7
3. Acyclovir (Zovirax) — 9
4. Albendazole (Albenza) — 11
5. Albuterol (ProAir, Ventolin, Proventil) — 13
6. Amoxicillin (Amoxil) — 15
7. Amoxicillin/Clavulanate (Augmentin) — 17
8. Amphetamine/Dextroamphetamine (Adderall) — 19
9. Amphotericin B (Fungizone) — 21
10. Antipyrine/Benzocaine (A/B Otic) — 23
11. Aripiprazole (Abilify) — 25
12. Atomoxetine (Strattera) — 27
13. Azithromycin (Zithromax) — 29
14. Budesonide (Pulmicort) — 31
15. Budesonide/Formoterol (Symbicort) — 33
16. Cefdinir (Omnicef) — 35
17. Cefixime (Suprax) — 37
18. Cefuroxime Axetil (Ceftin) — 39
19. Cephalexin (Keflex) — 41
20. Cetirizine (Zyrtec) — 43

| | | |
|---|---|---|
| 21. | Ceftriaxone (Rocephin) | 45 |
| 22. | Ciprofloxacin/Dexamethasone Otic (Ciprodex) | 47 |
| 23. | Clindamycin (Cleocin) | 49 |
| 24. | Clonidine (Kapvay) | 51 |
| 25. | Clotrimazole (Lotrimin) | 53 |
| 26. | DTaP Vaccine (Daptacel, Infanrix) | 55 |
| 27. | Desmopressin (DDAVP) | 57 |
| 28. | Dexamethasone (Decadron) | 59 |
| 29. | Dexmethylphenidate (Focalin) | 61 |
| 30. | Dextromethorphan (Delsym) | 63 |
| 31. | Diazepam Rectal Gel (Diastat) | 65 |
| 32. | Diphenhydramine (Benadryl) | 67 |
| 33. | Diphenhydramine Injection (Benadryl Injection) | 69 |
| 34. | Docusate Sodium (Colace) | 71 |
| 35. | Electrolyte Oral Solution (Pedialyte) | 73 |
| 36. | Epinephrine (EpiPen, Auvi-Q) | 75 |
| 37. | Erythromycin Ophthalmic Ointment (Ilotycin) | 77 |
| 38. | Famotidine (Pepcid) | 79 |
| 39. | Ferrous Sulfate | 81 |
| 40. | Fexofenadine (Allegra) | 83 |
| 41. | Fluoxetine (Prozac) | 85 |
| 42. | Fluconazole (Diflucan) | 87 |
| 43. | Fluticasone (Flovent) | 89 |
| 44. | Fluticasone Nasal (Flonase) | 91 |
| 45. | Fluticasone/Salmeterol (Advair) | 93 |
| 46. | Furosemide (Lasix) | 95 |
| 47. | Glycerin Suppositories | 97 |
| 48. | Guaifenesin (Mucinex) | 99 |

| | | |
|---|---|---|
| 49. | Guanfacine (Intuniv) | 101 |
| 50. | Hepatitis B Vaccine | 103 |
| 51. | Hydrochlorothiazide (HCTZ) | 105 |
| 52. | Hydrocortisone Cream (Cortizone) | 107 |
| 53. | Hydroxyzine (Atarax, Vistaril) | 109 |
| 54. | Ibuprofen (Advil, Motrin) | 111 |
| 55. | Influenza Vaccine (Fluzone – Injection, FluMist – Nasal Spray) | 113 |
| 56. | Insulin (Humulin, Novolog, Lantus) | 115 |
| 57. | Lactulose (Generlac) | 117 |
| 58. | Lamotrigine (Lamictal) | 119 |
| 59. | Levalbuterol (Xopenex) | 121 |
| 60. | Levetiracetam (Keppra) | 123 |
| 61. | Levothyroxine (Synthroid) | 125 |
| 62. | Lisdexamfetamine (Vyvanse) | 127 |
| 63. | Loperamide (Imodium) | 129 |
| 64. | Loratadine (Claritin) | 131 |
| 65. | MMR Vaccine (M-M-R II) | 133 |
| 66. | Mebendazole (Emverm) | 135 |
| 67. | Melatonin | 137 |
| 68. | Methotrexate | 139 |
| 69. | Methylphenidate (Ritalin, Concerta, Metadate) | 141 |
| 70. | Metronidazole (Flagyl) | 143 |
| 71. | Midazolam (Versed) | 145 |
| 72. | Mometasone Nasal (Nasonex) | 147 |
| 73. | Montelukast (Singulair) | 149 |
| 74. | Multivitamin with Iron (Poly-Vi-Sol) | 151 |
| 75. | Mupirocin (Bactroban) | 153 |
| 76. | Nitrofurantoin (Macrobid, Macrodantin) | 155 |

| | | |
|---|---|---|
| 77. | Nystatin (Mycostatin) | 157 |
| 78. | Ofloxacin Otic (Floxin Otic) | 159 |
| 79. | Omeprazole (Prilosec) | 161 |
| 80. | Ondansetron (Zofran) | 163 |
| 81. | Oseltamivir (Tamiflu) | 165 |
| 82. | Oxcarbazepine (Trileptal) | 167 |
| 83. | Penicillin V (Pen-Vee K) | 169 |
| 84. | Permethrin (Elimite, Nix) | 171 |
| 85. | Phenobarbital | 173 |
| 86. | Phenylephrine (Sudafed PE) | 175 |
| 87. | Pimecrolimus Cream (Elidel) | 177 |
| 88. | Pneumococcal Vaccine (Prevnar 13) | 179 |
| 89. | Polyethylene Glycol (MiraLAX) | 181 |
| 90. | Prednisolone (Orapred, Prelone) | 183 |
| 91. | Prednisolone Acetate Ophthalmic (Pred Forte) | 185 |
| 92. | Prednisone | 187 |
| 93. | Promethazine (Phenergan) | 189 |
| 94. | Pseudoephedrine (Sudafed) | 191 |
| 95. | Risperidone (Risperdal) | 193 |
| 96. | Senna (Senokot) | 195 |
| 97. | Sertraline (Zoloft) | 197 |
| 98. | Silver Sulfadiazine Cream (Silvadene) | 199 |
| 99. | Simethicone (Mylicon) | 201 |
| 100. | Sodium Chloride 0.9% IV | 203 |
| 101. | Sulfamethoxazole/Trimethoprim (Bactrim, Septra) | 205 |
| 102. | Tacrolimus Ointment (Protopic) | 207 |
| 103. | Tobramycin | 209 |
| 104. | Topical Lidocaine/Prilocaine (EMLA Cream) | 211 |

105. Triamcinolone Cream (Kenalog)     213

106. Trimethoprim/Sulfamethoxazole (Bactrim)     215

107. Valacyclovir (Valtrex)     217

108. Varicella Vaccine (Varivax)     219

109. Vitamin D3 (Cholecalciferol)     221

# WHY Made Easy Works

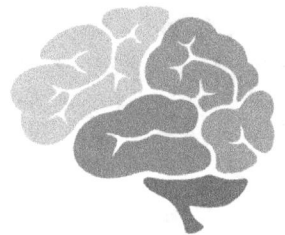

## Backed by Brain Science

Let's face it — nursing school can feel like trying to drink from a firehose. Between the jargon, the never-ending lists, and the sheer volume of information, it's easy to feel overwhelmed. That's exactly why the Made Easy series was born: to make the hard stuff stick without frying your brain. And while it might look fun and playful on the outside (hello, rhymes!), it's all built on rock-solid research from the nerdy world of educational psychology.

## 1. COGNITIVE LOAD THEORY

First up: Cognitive Load Theory. Fancy name, simple idea — your brain can only handle so much at once. When materials are too dense or packed with fluff, your working memory taps out. Educational psychologist John Sweller figured this out, and we took notes. That's why our poems give you the essentials only, in small, memorable doses. Less clutter, more clarity. (Sweller, 1988; Clark et al., 2006)

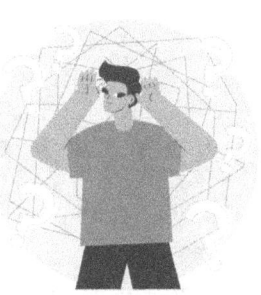

## 2. DUAL CODING THEORY

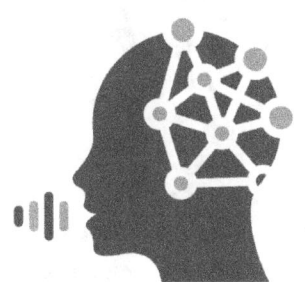

Then there's Dual Coding Theory, brought to us by Allan Paivio. He discovered that we remember things better when we learn them through both words and visuals. Our poems lean into this by using rhyme and rhythm to boost verbal memory — and bolded key terms, color coding, and clean formatting to give your visual brain a treat. Two paths to your brain = double the retention. (Paivio, 1986; Mayer, 2009)

## 3. ADVANCE ORGANIZERS

Psychologist David Ausubel believed that when we know how new info fits into what we already know, we learn faster. That's the beauty of our repeatable poem structure. Once you get the hang of the format, your brain relaxes — and focuses on what actually matters: the content. Think of it like a familiar playlist for your mind. (Ausubel, 1960)

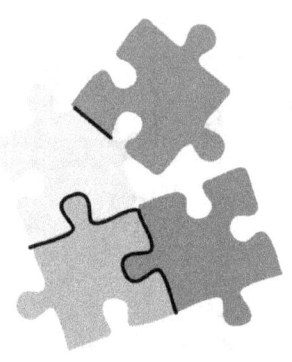

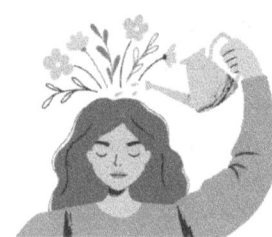

## 4. MICROLEARNING

Our poems are also bite-sized by design, and that's no accident. Welcome to the world of microlearning — the idea that small, focused learning units are easier to digest and retain. This is a game-changer for busy, burnt-out students. Instead of cramming for hours, you can study just one medication, one skill, or one critical concept at a time. Snack-sized studying with full-course impact. (Hug, 2005; van den Berg & van den Berg, 2021)

## 5. SPACED REPETITION & RETRIEVAL PRACTICE

Last but definitely not least: spaced repetition and retrieval practice. These two learning powerhouses have proven time and again that the more often you recall information over time, the longer you'll remember it. Our poems are made for this. Easy to reread, perfect for flashcards, and fun enough to come back to (yes, we admitted it). Rinse and repeat — and retain. (Dunlosky et al., 2013)

So, yes — this method might look different than your typical textbook grind. That's the point. It's effective on purpose. Because learning tough topics shouldn't feel impossible. It should feel doable. Even a little fun. And with Made Easy, it totally is.

# Read it. Rhyme it. Remember it.

That's the Made Easy Method—a simple but powerful approach to mastering complex nursing material.

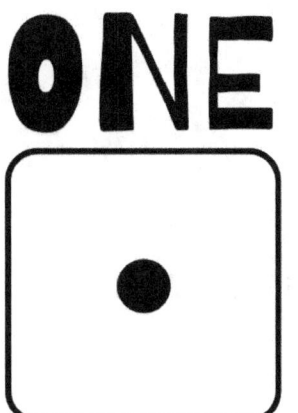

## THIS ISN'T REGULAR POETRY— IT'S PURPOSEFUL

These poems weren't made to be skimmed or read once.
They're built for memory. They're built for you.

They might feel dense at first. You might pause. That's okay.
You're supposed to wrestle with the words.
It's in that wrestling—the rereading, the out-loud reciting, the highlighting—that retention starts to kick in.

Let the rhythm do the heavy lifting.
Rhyme and repetition are memory's best friends.
This poetry is built for practice, not perfection.

## COLOR-CODE FOR CLARITY

To help you organize and absorb the content, we recommend using a color-coded system while you read.

Highlight or mark up key details with consistent colors for:

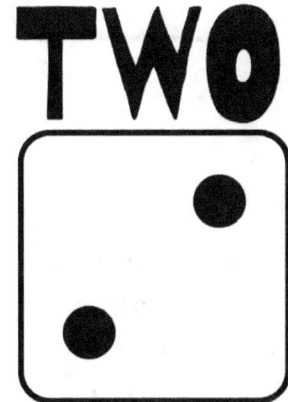

- 🟦 Drug Classification & Names
- 🟦 Mechanism of Action
- ⬜ Indications
- 🟦 Side Effects & Adverse Reactions
- 🟦 Nursing Considerations
- ◊ Monitoring Requirements
- 🟦 Patient & Caregiver Teaching Points
- ⬤ Black Box Warnings
- ⬜ Pediatric Considerations
- ⬤ Drug Interactions

When you revisit the poem, your highlights will guide your recall and make review sessions faster and easier.

# THREE

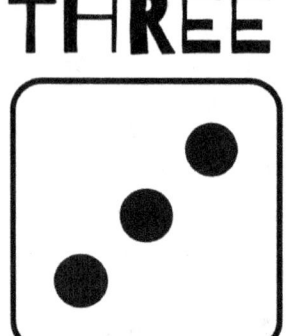

## TEST WHAT YOU KNOW

After each section, you'll find a QR code that takes you straight to a short NCLEX-style quiz hosted in Google Forms. These aren't just random practice questions — they're carefully crafted to test the most important takeaways from what you just read. But the real magic? <u>The rationales.</u> Whether you get the answer right or wrong, the quiz walks you through the why. Understanding the reasoning behind each answer helps you think like a nurse, not just a test-taker.

It's not about memorizing — it's about making connections, strengthening critical thinking, and applying your knowledge in real clinical scenarios. So take your time, review the rationales, and let them guide you from confusion to clarity.

# Acetaminophen (Tylenol)

*Non-opioid Analgesic; Antipyretic*

When **fevers run high** or **little ones ache**,
Acetaminophen's what we often will take.
It's gentle and trusted for **pain** that's mild,
A go-to choice for a **sick little child**.
It works in the brain, not the sites of the sore,
By **blocking prostaglandins**—but just at the core.
No bleeding risk like NSAIDs bring,
No tummy upset or stomach sting.

It helps with the **fever**, it **eases the pain**,
When teething or earaches come back again.
Given **by mouth** or sometimes **rectally**,
It's **safe when dosed carefully**, predictably.
But dose it with caution—**too much can harm**,
The **liver's at risk**, so raise the alarm
If mom gives a double, or dad grabs the cup,
Not knowing they've added too much syrup.

**Side effects** are rare, but don't dismiss—
**Hepatotoxicity** tops the list.

Watch for signs like **nausea** or skin that's **yellow**,
Or if they're unusually sleepy or mellow.
Check all the labels on what they ingest,
Cough syrups and combos—it's a sneaky guest.
**Teach parents** to measure with tools that are right,
Not spoons from the drawer in the middle of night.

Keep doses based on **weight, not age**,
Follow the guidelines, page by page.
And never give more than what's set in the day,
Or risk pushing the liver too far in the fray.
There's **no black box warning**, but still take care,
Acetaminophen needs awareness and flair.
It's a helpful tool in the nurse's cart—
But **education and dosing** play the biggest part.

# Ciprofloxacin Ophthalmic (Ciloxan)

*https://docs.google.com/forms/d/e/1FAIpQLSf0At2w58dxRLPmy592GRcz3N9k8ecbQ-lxPk99ViGYhdC6Vw/viewform?usp=header*

When **eyes turn red** and start to swell,
And **crusty discharge** starts to tell,
**Ciloxan** helps clear what's gone awry,
With **ciprofloxacin**—a drop for the eye.
It's part of the **fluoroquinolone crew**,
And **kills bacteria** that cloud the view.
It blocks DNA from copying right,
So the bugs can't grow in the soft eye light.

It's used for **pink eye** and **corneal scrape**,
To help infections **heal and reshape**.
**Drops or ointment**, several times a day,
But taper it down once symptoms give way.
**Burning** or **stinging** might briefly show,
Right when the drop starts to flow.
But it passes quick, and most won't mind,
As the eye begins to feel more kind.

Watch for **white patches** or any haze,

Signs of a **superinfection** in rare displays.

And though systemic effects are few,

Teach **clean technique** for parents to do.

Don't touch the tip to lashes or skin,

Or germs might sneak right back in.

Use **one bottle per child**, if both are ill,

To avoid spreading bugs against your will.

No **black box warning**, but still be smart—

**Allergic reactions** can sometimes start.

And if the eye gets worse, not better,

Call the doc—don't just write a letter.

Ciloxan's a helper for bacterial eyes,

Bringing **relief**, **clarity**, and fewer cries.

With careful drops and nursing support,

It helps those little peepers heal and report.

# Acyclovir (Zovirax)

*Antiviral Agent*

When **herpes** or **chickenpox** come into play,

**Acyclovir** helps chase the virus away.

From cold sores to shingles and spots on the skin,

It **slows viral growth** but won't fully win.

It doesn't cure—it's not magic, you see,

But it **shortens the flare-ups** and helps them break free.

It stops the virus from copying fast,

So symptoms improve, and rashes don't last.

It's used for **HSV**, **varicella** too,

In **kids who are high-risk** or breaking out new.

It might be **IV**, or **oral with food**,

Just be sure hydration is properly viewed.

It's gentle, but still, there are things to watch out,

Like **GI upset**, or a rash that may sprout.

**Headache**, **fatigue**, or a little confusion,

Could hint at a rare **renal intrusion**.

The **kidneys** must process this med with great care,

So **monitor urine** and labs with a stare.

Watch for **crystals** forming—hydrate them well,
Or risk **nephrotoxicity** that's hard to quell.
Teach parents it won't make the virus just go,
But it helps with **less pain** and a faster flow.
Start it **as soon as symptoms appear**,
For the best effect—it's crystal clear.

Remind them the virus can still be passed,
So **hand-washing**, **gloves**, and caution must last.
And **even if lesions begin to fade**,
Stay mindful—**contagion** hasn't fully decayed.
There's **no black box warning**, but don't let that sway—
This med needs **hydration** and labs on the way.
Zovirax is steady, a virus-fighting friend,
But nursing support makes the care truly blend.

# Albendazole (Albenza)

*Anthelmintic; Antiparasitic*

When **worms** invade from head to toe,
**Albendazole** helps make them go.
It's used when kids have **pinworms**, **hook**, or **tape**,
Or other invaders they can't escape.
It stops the worm's **tubulin track**,
So cells can't divide—they can't bounce back.
They **starve and die**, no room to thrive,
While the child feels better and more alive.

It's **chewed or swallowed**, sometimes with fat,
To help absorption—remember that!
**With food** is key, especially a meal,
For better results and a stronger heal.
It's **well-tolerated**, but there still may be,
**GI upset** or a **headache spree**.
**Elevated liver enzymes** can rise,
So labs are needed—be medically wise.

In **longer treatments**, check blood counts too,
For **low platelets** or **WBCs** sneaking through.

**Visual changes** or rash? Report right away.
Though rare, side effects can have their say.
**Pregnancy tests** if the patient can bear,
Because this med needs precaution and care.
**Teaching** includes washing hands and toys,
And treating the household—**girls and boys**.

Teach parents worms love to spread with ease,
So clean the sheets and scrub those knees.
Clip the nails and bleach the floor—
They'll thank you when the worms are no more.
There's **no black box**, but still play smart,
With **monitoring labs** right from the start.
Albendazole's a worm-fighting champ,
But nurses ensure it's a safe, clean camp.

# Albuterol (ProAir, Ventolin, Proventil)

*Short-Acting Beta-2 Agonist (SABA)*

When breathing is tight and wheezing won't quit,
**Albuterol** steps in to help airways split.
It **relaxes smooth muscles**, opens the way,
So **bronchioles widen**, and breath finds its stay.
It's the **rescue med** when asthma flares,
For coughs, for wheezing, for panic stares.
**Inhaler**, **nebulizer**, or sometimes **oral**,
But **inhaled** is fastest—clinical moral.

It **acts on beta-2**, lungs more than heart,
But **tachycardia** still can sometimes start.
**Shaky hands, nervousness, jittery feels**,
Are normal effects as the airway heals.
Too much? Then tremors, or heart rates that race,
So always **teach parents** to dose with grace.
**Use a spacer** if the kid is small,
To get the full dose—not just a wall.

**Wait 1-2 minutes between puffs** that are paired,

And rinse the mouth if **steroids** are shared.

Though **albuterol alone** won't coat or stick,

The rinse still helps—it's a good habit to pick.

Keep track of how often the rescue is used,

Too frequent? Then asthma's being abused.

That's a sign the plan needs a tweak or a test,

Maybe a **controller** to help them rest.

**Monitor lungs** before and after the med,

**Respiratory rate**, and how well they're fed.

If they're too tired to eat or play,

That's a clue the lungs aren't okay.

There's **no black box**, but don't play it light—

Frequent reliance means something's not right.

Used right, it's a breath of relief in a storm,

Bringing **lungs back to life** and **breathing to norm**.

# Amoxicillin (Amoxil)

*Aminopenicillin Antibiotic*

For **earaches**, **throat pain**, or a **runny green nose**,
**Amoxicillin** is how healing goes.
It's a **penicillin**, gentle yet strong,
Knocking out bugs that don't belong.
It stops them from **building their cell wall shell**,
So bacteria burst—and don't do well.
Great for **strep**, **otitis**, **sinus pain**,
And even **dental abscess** or **UTI strain**.

But this med comes with some common flair—
Like **diarrhea** that needs gentle care.
A bit of a rash can sometimes show,
Especially with viruses hiding below.
Some kids get **nausea**, a **tummy upset**,
So **take it with food**, that's your best bet.
And always finish the full round through,
Even if symptoms start to undo.

Watch for signs of **allergy fast**—
**Hives**, **swelling**, or if **breathing won't last**.

If there's **anaphylaxis**, it's urgent and dire,
Stop the med, give **epi**, call for fire.
**Renal function** matters, adjust if it's low,
And with **mononucleosis**, rash might show.
If a rash appears but they're not in distress,
It might not mean allergy—just viral mess.

Teach parents to measure—not guess or pour,
No kitchen spoons—use the ones from the store.
Shake the bottle if it's liquid inside,
And **refrigerate** it—unless otherwise specified.
There's **no black box**, but be aware,
**Superinfections** may surface with flare.
Like **yeast** or **C. diff** when good bugs fall—
So watch for new symptoms and catch them all.

# Amoxicillin/Clavulanate (Augmentin)

*Aminopenicillin + Beta-Lactamase Inhibitor*

When plain old **amoxicillin** won't do,
We call on **Augmentin** to help push through.
It's got **clavulanate**, a clever sidekick,
That stops beta-lactamase from doing its trick.
Some bugs fight back, breaking meds apart,
But **clavulanate** blocks them right from the start.
Together they punch through tougher strains,
Like **resistant sinus bugs**, **lungs**, or **glands** in pain.

It's used for **earaches**, **strep**, and **bronchitis** too,
Even **UTIs** when other drugs won't do.
A true upgrade when plain meds flop—
It gives stubborn infections a reason to stop.
But watch that **GI**—it's a little intense,
**Diarrhea** and **nausea** make common sense.
So always give it **with food in the belly**,
To keep it from bubbling like wobbly jelly.

It may cause a **rash**, like its cousin before,

And rare are the cases where **liver labs soar**.

An **allergic reaction** is still a concern,

So watch for those **hives** or **wheezes that burn**.

**Shake the bottle** if it's liquid they take,

And **keep it chilled** in the fridge for its sake.

Measure it right—no guessing allowed,

And **finish the course**, make your doctor proud.

**Yeast infections** can sneak in late,

So check for **diaper rash** or things that irritate.

It can throw off the gut and all its guests,

So watch for **C. diff** or GI unrest.

No **black box warning**, but don't play loose,

This med is strong—**respect its use**.

Augmentin fights with a dual sword swing,

To help little ones heal from almost anything.

# Amphetamine/Dextroamphetamine (Adderall)

*Central Nervous System Stimulant*

For focus that drifts or minds that roam,
**Adderall** helps bring attention home.
A mix of two stimulants working as one,
To help kids with **ADHD** get things done.
It boosts up **dopamine** and **norepinephrine**,
So the brain can **filter** and **lock things in**.
Improves **attention**, **impulse**, and **drive**,
Helps kids with **hyperactivity thrive**.

Given **by mouth**, and often **each day**,
But always in **morning**—not evening, okay?
It can make **bedtime battles** a real tough fight,
So avoid giving **late into night**.
Side effects can be tough to ignore—
Like **loss of appetite**, eating much less than before.
**Stomachaches, headaches,** and **trouble at rest**,
**Mood swings** or **jitters** may also suggest.

It may raise the **heart rate** or **blood pressure too**,
So **cardiac history** must be reviewed.
Some kids may seem quiet or oddly flat,
So monitor **mood** and behavior at that.
This med is **controlled**, so handle with care,
**Locked up at home**, with strict dosing there.
**No double-dosing** if one's ever missed—
Just skip and resume, keep it off the twist.

**Growth can slow**, so track their height,
And **weight each visit** to keep things right.
Long-term use means **labs and checks**,
To keep a watch on side effect specs.
Teach parents this isn't a magic fix,
It's part of a full ADHD mix—
With **structure**, **routine**, and **school support**,
So kids stay strong in every report.

There's **no black box** for children per se,
But adults face risks if it's **misused in any way**.
So screen for **abuse**, and follow with grace,
This med needs **respect** in every case.

# Amphotericin B (Fungizone)
*Antifungal (Polyene Class)*

When **fungal infections** go deep and wild,
**Amphotericin B** is given to the child.
For **systemic mycoses**, it's strong and bold,
But oh—this med is a handful to hold.
It pokes through the **fungal cell membrane wall**,
Binding to **ergosterol** to make it fall.
It leaks out the insides, the fungus will die,
But the **side effects** might make you sigh.

Nicknamed "**Amphoterrible**," nurses know why—
**Chills**, **fever**, and **rigors** can quickly fly.
**Hypotension**, **nephrotoxicity**, too,
And **hypokalemia** may be breaking through.
Given **IV only**—and very slow,
In a **central line** if you can go.
Premedicate with **Tylenol**, **Benadryl**, and such,
To ease the **infusion reaction** punch.

It's used for **cryptococcus**, **candida**, and more,
Especially in **immunocompromised** cases we store.

But never take it lightly—it needs trained eyes,
With labs and vitals checked for surprise.
**Monitor kidneys**, the **BUN and creatinine**,
And **daily weights** to catch fluid within.
Check **electrolytes**, especially **K** and **Mg**,
Supplement as needed so levels don't sag.

Teach parents why it's not taken by mouth,
And that side effects may head slightly south.
Reassure that reactions can be controlled,
When given with planning and nursing bold.
There's **no black box**, but it carries weight,
So **monitor labs** and don't medicate late.
It's life-saving, yes—but also intense,
A **last-line antifungal** in the right defense.

# Antipyrine/Benzocaine (A/B Otic)

*Otic Analgesic and Anesthetic Combo*

When **earaches** scream and tears are loud,
**A/B Otic** can calm the crowd.
It's a blend of **benzocaine** to numb the sting,
And **antipyrine** to ease the pain it brings.
It doesn't cure infection inside,
But it **soothes the canal** where the pain may hide.
A **topical drop**, not swallowed at all,
Just a few in the ear—no need to call.

Used for **otitis media** when pressure is tight,
To help little ones **rest through the night**.
The warmth can comfort, the sting will fade,
A temporary fix that's carefully made.
It may cause **mild redness** or **irritation**,
So monitor closely with each application.
And if there's a **ruptured drum**, beware—
This med should **never** be placed in there.

Teach parents to **warm the bottle by hand**,
Then gently **pull the ear** just as planned.

For kids under three, pull **down and back**,

To help the drops follow the proper track.

Keep it **clean**—no sharing, no tip in the ear,

Just drop it in gently, then comfort is near.

**Don't use for long**, it's short-term relief,

And **antibiotics** may be needed for grief.

There's **no black box**, but caution is wise—

Especially if symptoms begin to rise.

A/B Otic soothes but won't make it gone,

So **follow-up care** must still carry on.

# Aripiprazole (Abilify)

*Atypical Antipsychotic*

When moods are swinging or voices appear,
**Abilify** helps make things clear.
It's used for **bipolar**, **autism**, and **psychosis**, too,
Even **irritability** when nothing else will do.
It works in the brain on **dopamine flow**,
A **partial agonist**—fast, but slow.
It balances **dopamine** and **serotonin's ride**,
To calm the storm and clear the tide.

It's given by **mouth**, sometimes as a **shot**,
Atypical, yes—but side effects? A lot.
May cause **insomnia**, or make kids feel tired,
Sometimes they're restless, sometimes they're wired.
Watch for **weight gain**, though usually light,
And **akathisia**—that jittery fight.
Some get **tremors**, **dizzy**, or **numb**,
While others feel flat or emotionally numb.

**Monitor mood**—especially dark,
As suicidal thinking can leave its mark.

There's a **black box warning** for **youth at risk**,

So assess mental status—not just a checklist.

Check **blood sugar** and **lipids**, too,

As metabolic changes may wander through.

Watch **liver enzymes**, and **EPS signs**,

And always screen for **prolonged QT lines**.

Teach families it doesn't work in a day,

And **compliance is key** to keep symptoms at bay.

**No alcohol**, avoid OTC meds with care,

And **don't stop suddenly**—that's never fair.

This med supports, but it won't cure,

So therapy and love must also endure.

With careful watching and plans that align,

**Abilify** helps young minds realign.

# Atomoxetine (Strattera)

*Selective Norepinephrine Reuptake Inhibitor (NRI)*

When focus is foggy and thoughts run free,
**Strattera** helps with **ADHD**.
It's not a stimulant, but still sharp and wise,
A non-controlled option that helps kids rise.
It works by **blocking norepinephrine's fall**,
So more stays active to **focus them all**.
It's slow to start—but steady and true,
Building effects over a week or two.

**No highs, no crashes**, no jittery feels,
But sometimes brings its own set of deals.
**Nausea, fatigue**, and a dry little mouth,
And **decreased appetite**—heading south.
Mood may dip, so check in tight—
**Suicidal thoughts** can creep in at night.
There's a **black box warning** for mental decline,
So monitor closely for any sign.

Check **liver labs**, though it's rare they rise,
Watch **BP**, **heart rate**, and teary eyes.

Some may get **urinary hesitation**,
Or feel some mood **dysregulation**.
It's taken by mouth, once daily with care,
**Not crushed or split**—swallow it there.
And **don't stop suddenly** without the plan,
It needs a taper, a guiding hand.

No abuse risk like others might show,
So **parents may prefer** it over the go-go.
But it's slower—needs time, like a tree to grow,
So patience and structure help progress flow.
It's **not for everyone**, but when it's the key,
It can help a young mind **focus and be**.
With check-ins, support, and nursing insight,
Strattera can help their day feel right.

# Azithromycin (Zithromax)

*Macrolide Antibiotic*

For **earaches**, **strep**, or a **chesty cough**,
**Zithromax** helps to knock germs off.
It's part of the **macrolide** family tree,
With a long half-life and dosing ease.
It stops bacteria from making their chain,
By **blocking ribosomes** in the protein lane.
No protein? No life? The bacteria fall—
That's how **azithro** outsmarts them all.

A favorite for **kids who can't do penicillin**,
It's often a backup when rashes are chillin'.
From **pneumonia**, to **strep**, to **pink eye**, too,
It's a versatile med in the nurse's crew.
Once a day for **three to five**,
The shorter course helps parents survive.
But don't let the shortness fool the plan—
**Finish it all**—yes, that's the stand!

**GI upset** is the most common side,
**Nausea**, maybe **diarrhea**, along for the ride.

It can also **prolong the QT**,

So check their **heart rhythm** if there's a history.

Rarely, the **liver** might not feel great,

So check **ALT**, **AST**, and evaluate.

**Rash? Hives?** Could be allergy's call—

Stop the med and report it all.

No **black box warning**, but still go slow,

When heart or liver risks may show.

Teach parents to give it on time, not late,

And **shake the suspension** before they medicate.

Avoid **antacids** within a span,

Of dosing time—it's part of the plan.

And watch for **superinfections** if things don't improve,

Or yeast infections that might make a move.

Zithromax is strong with a kid-friendly pace,

But nursing support helps it win the race.

# Budesonide (Pulmicort)

*Inhaled Corticosteroid*

When airways are tight and swelling won't quit,
**Pulmicort** helps them breathe a bit.
It's not a rescue—but more of a shield,
To **quiet the lungs** and help them heal.
A **steroid** inhaled to reduce the flame,
Of asthma's swelling and mucus game.
It cuts down **inflammation** deep inside,
So breathing improves and symptoms subside.

It's used in **daily asthma control** for kids,
To stop flare-ups before they hit the skids.
Given by **neb** or **Flexhaler puff**,
With regular use—not just when it's tough.
It doesn't bring jitter or racing hearts,
But needs time and **routine** to do its part.
**Not a rescue**—that's albuterol's job,
Pulmicort's slow, but steady on the mob.

It may cause a **sore throat** or a **hoarse sound**,
And sometimes a **cough** when it swirls around.

The most important teaching point? Clear—
**Rinse the mouth after every use, my dear!**
That helps prevent **oral thrush**, you see,
A white, patchy fungal enemy.
**Growth delays** are rare, but can appear,
So track their **height and weight each year.**

No **black box warning**, but still take care,
It's a long-term med, so nurses beware.
Watch for signs that asthma's flared,
And make sure parents are well-prepared.
Teach them this med is part of the base,
Not for panic, but for **steady grace**.
Pulmicort helps keep the airways wide,
With calm lungs and peace inside.

# Budesonide/Formoterol (Symbicort)

*Inhaled Corticosteroid + Long-Acting Beta-2 Agonist (LABA)*

When asthma's control starts slipping away,
**Symbicort** steps in to save the day.
A **combo med** with a dual attack,
To **calm inflammation** and **hold flare-ups back**.
**Budesonide** tames the swollen airways tight,
While **Formoterol** helps them open just right.
A **steroid and bronchodilator** blend,
For **maintenance use**—not rescue, my friend.

It's taken **twice daily**, every day,
To keep those symptoms well at bay.
For kids with **asthma** that won't behave,
It's a **controller med** their lungs will crave.
**Not for sudden wheezing**, not for a scare,
That's **albuterol's job** in urgent air.
This one works best when used with care,
And taken **consistently**, not on a dare.

It may cause **headache**, or **hoarseness**, too,
And sometimes a **shaky or jittery view**.
But rinse the mouth out after each puff,
To stop **oral thrush** from getting rough.
**Formoterol** can raise **heart rate** a bit,
So check for **palpitations** that just don't quit.
Also assess for **chest pain** or **restless sleep**,
Especially in children who feel it deep.

There's a **black box warning** for LABAs alone—
They must be used with steroids as shown.
But in **Symbicort**, they're safely paired,
As long as the plan is clearly shared.
Teach families the difference between each med,
One for **rescue**, one to **keep symptoms ahead**.
**Shake before use**, then **inhale it slow**,
And teach them the steps so they confidently know.

Symbicort's power is steady and strong,
When asthma control has struggled too long.
It's not a cure, but with structure and care,
It gives little lungs more room for air.

# Cefdinir (Omnicef)

*Third-Generation Cephalosporin Antibiotic*

When the sniffles turn sour or the cough won't rest,
**Omnicef** steps up and handles the test.
A **cephalosporin**, third-gen and bright,
It fights off the bugs that don't go down light.
From **ear infections** to **sinus pain**,
To **bronchitis**, **strep**, and even a **strain**
Of **mild skin infections**, it clears the way—
A tasty red syrup kids take each day.

It works by breaking the bug's strong wall,
So bacteria burst and take the fall.
A **bactericidal** with serious might,
But it needs the **full course** to win the fight.
Some kids get a **rash** or a **bit of the runs**,
**Diarrhea** is common in little ones.
Sometimes the **stool turns red or bold**,
But it's just the med—not blood, we're told.

It may upset the **tummy**, cause **nausea**, or gas,
So **give it with food** to help it pass.

Watch for signs of **allergy, itching, or hives**,
And rare reactions that threaten lives.
If there's a **penicillin allergy** in play,
Check with the doc before giving away.
There's **cross-reactivity**, just a trace,
But still worth caution—just in case.

**Shake the bottle**, refrigerate tight,
Unless the label says room temp's right.
Measure it properly—no guessing dose,
And **complete the course**, that matters most.
No **black box warning**, but don't overlook—
Watch for **yeast infections** that quietly took.
And **C. diff colitis**, while rare, is real,
So watch for **bloody stools** or how they feel.

Cefdinir's handy when kids get sick,
But **nurses and parents** must stay quick.
With care and calm, and dosing done right,
Omnicef helps infections take flight.

# Cefixime (Suprax)

*Third-Generation Cephalosporin Antibiotic*

When fevers rise and throats get sore,
And the earache knocks at the bedroom door,
**Suprax** is there with a gentle kick—
**Cefixime** helps get rid of it quick.
A **cephalosporin**, third-gen and neat,
It tackles infections that just won't retreat.
From **strep throat**, **earaches**, and **bronchitis bad**,
To **UTIs** in kids that make them sad.

It stops the bugs from building their wall,
So **cell lysis** happens—and down they fall.
A **bactericidal** agent, working with pride,
To clear out the mess bacteria hide.
It's usually **once a day**, which is nice,
For kids who aren't fans of dosing twice.
But side effects can come, so watch with care—
**Nausea**, **diarrhea**, floating in there.

**Rashes** may show or **itching begin**,
And that might mean allergy under the skin.

If there's a **penicillin allergy** in the chart,
There's a small chance cross-reaction could start.
Give it **with or without food**, just the same,
But **liquid form**? Shake before the game.
Use the right tool—**no spoons from the drawer**,
And keep going till there's **no doses more**.

Though it's rare, **C. diff** may follow behind,
So watch for stools that are out of line.
And signs of **yeast**—like rash or itch,
Might mean gut flora has made a switch.
There's **no black box**, but still keep track,
Of **fever**, **rash**, or behavior that's whack.
Suprax works best when given just right,
With **nursing eyes sharp** and **goals in sight**.

# Cefuroxime Axetil (Ceftin)

*Second-Generation Cephalosporin Antibiotic*

When germs dig deep and just won't quit,
**Ceftin** steps in with a cephalosporin hit.
It's **second-gen**, with a broader view,
Fighting **respiratory**, **ear**, and **urinary** too.
It breaks down the bug's **cell wall frame**,
So the bacteria burst—it's a losing game.
Used for **strep throat**, **otitis**, and **sinus blues**,
And even **skin infections** or a **tick-borne bruise**.

It comes as a **pill** or **suspension sweet**,
Though the taste can make it a bit of a feat.
**Give with food** to help it digest,
And **shake well** so each dose is the best.
**Side effects** may cause some mess—
Like **diarrhea**, **nausea**, or general distress.
Some kids get a **rash**, or **hives that appear**,
So watch for allergy—keep that clear.

And if they've had **penicillin before**,
Ask if there's allergy you shouldn't ignore.

There's some **cross-sensitivity**, just in case,

So double-check the med's safe in that space.

Teach parents: complete the course!

Even if symptoms take a better course.

Skipping or quitting too early might

Let sneaky bacteria reignite.

It rarely can lead to **yeast overgrowth**,

Or **C. diff colitis** (but not in most).

So monitor stools and diapered skin,

And report new symptoms once they begin.

No **black box warning**, but caution still,

With proper dosing and nursing skill.

Ceftin helps when the bugs dig in—

But **your teaching and tracking** help patients win.

# Cephalexin (Keflex)

*First-Generation Cephalosporin Antibiotic*

For **earaches**, **strep**, or a **rash that's red**,
**Keflex** clears the path where the germs have spread.
A **first-gen cephalosporin** tried and true,
It's gentle for kids, but tough on the flu—
Well… not the virus, but bacterial foes,
Like **strep skin infections** and **UTI woes**.

It **stops cell walls** from building strong,
So **bacteria burst** when they don't belong.
It's **bactericidal**, with solid might,
Given **by mouth**—day or night.
Dosed **two to four times** depending on case,
So teach parents to **keep a steady pace**.
And remind them: **don't skip, don't stop**,
Or the infection might circle back on top.

Side effects? Mostly **GI distress**,
Like **diarrhea**, **cramps**, or a bit of a mess.
Some may get **rash**, or an **itchy sign**,
So check for **allergy**, especially with time.

If there's a **penicillin allergy** on the chart,
Ask more questions before you start.
There's a **small cross-reaction** that could arise,
So don't let that slip under nursing eyes.

No **black box warning**, but yeast may bloom,
So watch for **oral thrush** or **diaper room**.
Rare but real: **C. diff** could appear,
If diarrhea is bad or smells weird and severe.
Give with or without food—it's flexible that way,
But **food may help** if the tummy won't stay.
And always remind: **Shake if it's liquid**,
And **measure it right**, not "just a little bit."
Keflex is classic, a nurse's old friend,
But your guidance ensures a healthy end.

# Cetirizine (Zyrtec)

*Second-Generation Antihistamine*

When noses drip and **eyes start to itch**,
And **seasonal sneezing** flips the switch,
**Zyrtec** helps calm the allergy tide,
With **cetirizine** working from the inside.
It's a **second-gen antihistamine**, smooth and clean,
So it **won't make kids as drowsy** as the first-gens seen.
It blocks **H1 receptors** to stop the sneeze,
And helps with **hives, rhinitis**, and **allergic wheeze**.

It's **once a day**, and can be sweet,
In **liquid or chewable** forms to eat.
It kicks in fast and lasts all day,
To keep histamine's chaos far away.
Side effects? There still might be,
A bit of **sleepiness** or **dry mouth spree**.
Maybe a **headache** or **tummy distress**,
But overall, it's well-tolerated—less stress.

Teach parents it's not for cold or flu,
It's **allergy-related**—that's the cue.

And while it's **OTC**, dosing's key,

So go by the label and weight, not "maybe."

No **black box warning**, no major alarms,

But keep meds out of reach—**little hands cause harm**.

And if paired with **other antihistamines**,

There's risk of **overdose**, though rare it seems.

So when pollen's high or hives appear,

Zyrtec brings calm and helps things clear.

A steady friend in the allergy zone,

But **nursing wisdom** still sets the tone.

# Ceftriaxone (Rocephin)

*Third-Generation Cephalosporin Antibiotic*

When an infection runs deep and won't let go,
**Rocephin** steps in with a powerful blow.
A **third-gen cephalosporin**, strong and wide,
Fighting bugs that like to **systemically hide**.
It treats **pneumonia**, **meningitis**, **UTIs**, too,
**Sepsis**, **gonorrhea**, and **earaches** that brew.
Given **IM** or **IV**—not by mouth,
It works when infections are heading south.

It stops bacteria from building their shell,
So **cell walls break down**—they don't do well.
It's **bactericidal**, fast and tight,
With a **long half-life**, dosing once feels right.
But nurses know it can bring a sting,
**IM shots hurt**—so lidocaine's a thing.
Mix it right and warm the dose,
To make the jab a little less gross.

Watch for **allergic reactions**, especially rash,
Or signs of **anaphylaxis** that come in a flash.

And if they've had **penicillin trouble**,
This could still pop the same allergic bubble.
It may cause **diarrhea**, **nausea**, and more,
And **C. diff risk** comes knocking at the door.
**Bilirubin levels**? Check with care—
In **newborns**, Rocephin **isn't fair**.

Teach families about the **once-a-day ease**,
But also about **safety**, not just disease.
Watch for signs of **yeast**, or stool that's red,
And always **complete the course**, just as said.
There's **no black box**, but use it wise,
Especially in **neonates**, where danger lies.
Rocephin's a warrior when things get rough,
But **nurses make sure the care is enough**.

# Ciprofloxacin/Dexamethasone Otic (Ciprodex)

*Fluoroquinolone Antibiotic + Corticosteroid (Otic Drops)*

When ears are red and swollen with pain,
And **otitis externa** won't wane in the rain,
**Ciprodex** drops are the go-to plan—
A mix of two meds in one tiny can.
**Ciprofloxacin** fights off the bugs,
Kicking out **bacteria** hiding in plugs.
While **dexamethasone** steps in to tame,
The **inflammation** that's fueling the flame.

It's great for **swimmer's ear**, tender and sore,
And sometimes for **tubes** with drainage galore.
**Twice a day**, for seven to ten,
With comfort and healing returning again.
The drops may sting or feel a bit cold,
So **warm the bottle** in hand to hold.
Have them **lay on the side** and stay quite still,
For **five minutes flat**, or longer if they will.

Don't touch the tip to the ear or skin,

Or germs from the outside might sneak back in.

And never use if the **eardrum is torn**,

Unless the doctor's guidance is sworn.

Most side effects are mild at best—

Like a **bit of discomfort** or fullness in the chest.

But **hypersensitivity** can still occur,

So report **rash, itching**, or anything unsure.

No **black box warning**, but still proceed

With education and careful heed.

Teach parents to **gently clean the ear**,

But **never use Q-tips**—let that be clear!

Ciprodex brings relief where pain once throbbed,

A trusted tool in the nursing job.

With calm, clean hands and drops just right,

It helps those **tiny ears sleep through the night**.

# Clindamycin (Cleocin)

*Lincosamide Antibiotic*

When **staph or strep** won't go away,
And **penicillin** can't save the day,
**Cleocin** comes in, strong and lean,
That's **clindamycin**—sharp and clean.
It stops bacteria from making their chains,
By **blocking ribosomes** in cellular lanes.
A **bacteriostatic**—it halts the spread,
Helping the immune system fight ahead.

It's used for **skin infections**, big and small,
And **abscesses** that bubble or try to sprawl.
Also used for **dental bugs**,
And **bone infections** hiding in hugs.
It comes **oral**, **IV**, or **topical cream**,
But **bitter when swallowed**, so plan for the team.
**Take with food** if the tummy's upset,
Though absorption's best when the belly's set.

Side effects? **GI distress** is key—
**Nausea**, **cramps**, and **diarrhea spree**.

But here's the flag to raise up quick:
**C. diff colitis**—and it can be sick.
Watch for **bloody stools** or pain down low,
If those show up—**stop it and go**.
It's one of the meds most famous for
Triggering **C. diff** from gut flora war.

No **black box warning**, but caution high,
Especially when **multiple doses apply**.
Check for signs of **rash** or **itch**,
A **hypersensitive switch** may flip the switch.
Teach parents not to skip or share,
Even if **symptoms no longer flare**.
**Complete the course**, as always taught—
Or resistance is something that could be caught.

Clindamycin fights deep and wide,
But with **nurse support** right by the side.
When used with care and wisdom strong,
It helps clear up what's been wrong.

# Clonidine (Kapvay)

*Alpha-2 Adrenergic Agonist*

When **focus is fleeting** and sleep won't stay,
**Kapvay** helps smooth the night and day.
That's **clonidine**, a calming med,
That quiets the thoughts that race in the head.
It's not a stimulant, but still has might,
Used for **ADHD**, especially at night.
It **activates alpha-2 receptors** inside,
To lower **norepinephrine's wild ride**.

The result? A brain that's more at peace,
With **impulses lowered** and **movement decrease**.
It also treats **tics**, **anxiety**, **sleep**,
And helps **blood pressure** not run too deep.
But side effects? Let's name a few:
**Sedation**, **fatigue**, and feeling "blue."
**Dry mouth**, **constipation**, and **dizzy spells**,
**Low heart rate** is something nursing tells.

Take it **at night** if drowsiness hits,
And rise up slow—avoid those splits.

But if **stopped too fast**, beware the race—
**Rebound hypertension** can take its place.
So taper it slow, with guidance tight,
Never just end it overnight.
It comes in **tablets**, swallowed with care,
And **extended-release** for steady repair.

No **black box warning**, but watch that heart,
And monitor **BP** from the start.
Teach parents how to **check the dose**,
And to **never crush**—that part is close.
Clonidine's gentle, but firm in role,
To help a child feel calm and whole.
With nurse support and a watchful guide,
Kapvay can help the storms subside.

# Clotrimazole (Lotrimin)

*Topical Antifungal (Imidazole Class)*

When little feet itch or red rings grow,
**Lotrimin** steps in to stop the show.
**Clotrimazole** fights the fungal flair,
Whether on skin, or scalp, or somewhere bare.
It blocks the fungus from building strong,
By **breaking ergosterol** all along.
That **weakens the wall** of fungal cells,
Until they leak—and no longer dwell.

Used for **ringworm**, **athlete's foot**, and **yeast**,
And **diaper rashes** where fungus has feast.
Apply it **twice daily**, clean and dry,
And watch the redness start to die.
It's **topical only**, not meant for the mouth,
Don't put it inside or deep down south.
And never near eyes—if it gets in there,
Just rinse it gently with water and care.

Side effects? Usually **itch or burn**,
Where the cream goes on—that's your turn.

But most do well and heal up fine,

With just a little **daily time**.

**Teach parents**: even if it looks okay,

**Keep using it** through the full display.

Stopping too soon might make it return,

And that's a lesson we all must learn.

No **black box warning**, and safe when used right,

Just wash your hands after each fight.

Lotrimin's gentle, and works with grace,

To clear the fungus from its place.

# DTaP Vaccine (Daptacel, Infanrix)

*Diphtheria, Tetanus, and Acellular Pertussis Vaccine*

When babies grow strong and start their race,
**DTaP** helps guard them, just in case.
It's a combo shot, three in one,
To fight off danger before it's begun.
**Diphtheria**—a throat-clogging scare,
**Tetanus** from wounds that don't heal with care,
And **Pertussis**—that whooping cough cry,
DTaP protects so fewer kids die.

It's given **IM**, most often the thigh,
At **2, 4, 6 months**, as time goes by.
Boosters follow at **15–18 months** and four,
Then **Tdap** comes later when they're big and explore.
Side effects are usually small and brief—
Like **redness**, **swelling**, or crying in grief.
A **low-grade fever**, a **lump at the site**,
Or being a little more clingy at night.

But serious reactions are rare to see,
Like **high fever**, or **seizures**, or **fainting spree**.

So nurses watch and parents stay near,

For any strange symptoms that may appear.

**Teach parents**: this shot doesn't mean they're done—

It's part of a **series**, not just one.

Comfort the child, use cuddles and care,

And offer some **Tylenol** if the fever is there.

It's not given with a **history of allergy**

To vaccine components—check carefully.

And not for those with a **past seizure scare**

Until the provider is fully aware.

No **black box warning**, but education is key,

To build vaccine trust in the whole family.

DTaP's a defender, one of the best,

Giving little immune systems a shield and a vest.

# Desmopressin (DDAVP)

*Synthetic Antidiuretic Hormone (ADH Analog)*

When kids keep peeing through the night,
Or can't hold water with all their might,
**DDAVP** can lend a hand—
**Desmopressin**, calm and planned.
It mimics **ADH** in the brain,
To help the **kidneys hold fluid** again.
Less urine made, more water kept,
So kids wake dry and parents slept.

Used for **bedwetting** in children who try,
Or **diabetes insipidus** when levels run dry.
Even **bleeding disorders** like mild vWD—
It boosts **factor VIII**, which helps the bleed.
Comes in **tabs**, **nasal spray**, or **IV drip**,
Depending on age, condition, and script.
But here's the warning every nurse must say:
Too much can take **sodium away**.

**Hyponatremia** is the biggest fear,
With **headaches**, **nausea**, and **mental unclear**.

So monitor **electrolytes**, especially **Na**,
And limit fluids in a thoughtful way.
**Daily weights** and **I&O**,
Track how much in and how much go.
Signs of **water intoxication** may rise—
So watch for confusion or puffy eyes.

It's well-tolerated when used with sense,
But teach with care and confidence.
Give **in the evening** if bedwetting's the cause,
And always follow the provider's laws.
No **black box warning**, but caution stands,
With **fluid restriction** in caring hands.
DDAVP can change a kid's day,
But **nursing support** clears the way.

# Dexamethasone (Decadron)

*Corticosteroid (Glucocorticoid)*

When **swelling**, **inflammation**, or **wheezing** appear,
**Decadron** steps in to make things clear.
It's a **glucocorticoid**, strong and fast,
To **calm immune storms** and help healing last.
It's used for **croup**, where that barky cough grows,
To shrink down the airway and let air flow.
Also given for **asthma**, **allergies**, **chemo side pain**,
And **brain swelling**, **nausea**, or trauma to the brain.

It lowers **cytokines**, cools the flame,
And helps the body get back in the game.
It's given **oral**, **IV**, **IM**—you choose,
Depending on what the child could lose.
But with its strength come side effects,
So nurses prepare and double-check.
**Mood swings**, **insomnia**, **stomach upset**,
And **increased blood sugar**—a frequent threat.

**Irritability** might come in fast,
Especially if given more than just one blast.

**Weight gain**, **puffy face**, or a **rosy glow**,

Can appear with use—so let parents know.

Watch out for **long-term use**, where risks grow deep,

Like **bone thinning**, or **growth delays** that creep.

And if stopped suddenly after steady use,

**Adrenal crisis** could cut loose.

**Tapering** is key if the dose runs long,

To keep that cortisol rhythm strong.

No **black box warning**, but still proceed

With patient teaching and nursing speed.

Teach to **give with food** to protect the gut,

And **track mood changes**, even if slight or abrupt.

Decadron helps when the body's in fight—

But your care ensures it's handled right.

# Dexmethylphenidate (Focalin)

*Central Nervous System Stimulant*

When **focus drifts** and thoughts run wild,
**Focalin** helps calm the scattered child.
It's a **stimulant med**, precise and lean,
A refined version of **methylphenidate's team**.
It boosts the brain with dopamine flow,
Helping **attention**, **impulse**, and **focus grow**.
Used for **ADHD** most every day,
To help kids learn, and work, and play.

It kicks in fast and doesn't delay,
So **morning doses** start the day.
There's **immediate** and **XR**, both in the game,
But **never crush**—the rules stay the same.
Side effects may tag along for the ride,
Like **decreased appetite**, or **nerves inside**.
**Stomachaches**, **headaches**, and **trouble at rest**,
**Mood shifts** or **tics**—though not in every test.

**Check height and weight** as kids may grow slow,
And track **blood pressure** before you go.

It may raise the **HR**, a bit too much,
So watch for **palpitations**, and stay in touch.
There's **no black box** just for the youth,
But misuse and abuse are a serious truth.
This med is **controlled**—keep safe and tight,
In a **locked-up spot** and out of sight.

**Teach parents** not to double the dose,
If one gets missed, just let it go.
And monitor closely for **mood or sleep**,
Because even small changes may run deep.
Focalin's sharp when used just right,
Helping kids shine and settle their flight.
With **nurse support** and a steady plan,
It helps young minds do all they can.

# Dextromethorphan (Delsym)

*Cough Suppressant (Antitussive)*

When **coughs won't quit** and kids can't rest,
**Delsym** helps the chest feel best.
With **dextromethorphan** leading the way,
It calms the urge to cough all day.
It works on the **brain's cough control zone**,
To quiet the reflex and soothe the tone.
Not for mucus, not for wet,
But for **dry, hacking coughs** you won't forget.

It's **non-opioid**, but still be wise—
Too much can lead to **weird highs**.
In large amounts it **acts like a hallucinogen**,
So keep it locked from curious kin.
Usually safe in the proper dose,
But **under age 4**? It's a no-go most.
**Pediatric use** should follow the guide,
And **combination products** should not be wide.

**Side effects** are gentle—maybe **nausea** or **dizzy**,
Some feel **drowsy**, others get **busy**.

And if the dose is way too high,
It may cause **confusion** or **euphoria's sky**.
Teach parents to **read the label well**,
Especially if multiple meds dwell.
This drug can **hide in cold and flu**,
So double-check what else they do.

There's **no black box**, but caution still,
Especially in teens with time to kill.
Used right, it's safe—and works with grace,
To help a child breathe in quiet space.

# Diazepam Rectal Gel (Diastat)

*Benzodiazepine; Anticonvulsant*

When **seizures strike** and won't let go,
**Diastat** helps to stop the show.
It's **diazepam**, in **rectal form**,
To calm the brain and quiet the storm.
Used in **status epilepticus** that won't break,
It gives the brain a needed brake.
For kids with seizures that go too long,
This rescue med is **fast and strong**.

It enhances **GABA's calming flow**,
To **slow down signals** that start the show.
It's not for daily use or flair—
But kept **on hand for urgent care**.
Given **rectally, pre-filled and sealed**,
With careful dosing that's clearly revealed.
**Parents are trained** to use it right,
To act in the middle of a seizure fight.

**Side effects** may follow the dose,
Like **sleepiness**, **wobble**, or **slow response** close.

**Respiratory depression** is rare but real,

So monitor breathing—it's part of the deal.

**Teach caregivers** to time the event,

And **call 911** if it's still intense.

Give one dose, and **don't repeat**,

Unless the doctor's plan is complete.

Check **age**, **weight**, and **tolerance build**,

Too much benzo use leaves the receptors chilled.

There's **no black box**, but warnings apply,

For misuse, sedation, and reasons why.

It's a lifeline drug in a little tube,

Helping kids get past the seizure rube.

With **clear education**, courage, and care,

Diastat works when seconds are rare.

# Diphenhydramine (Benadryl)

*First-Generation Antihistamine*

When **hives pop up** or **allergies flare**,
Benadryl is often right there.
It's **diphenhydramine**, old and well-known,
Blocking **histamine** so symptoms are shown the door and gone.
It works on the **H1 receptor path**,
To calm the itching, rash, or wrath.
Used for **allergies**, **stings**, and **sneezes**, too,
Even **motion sickness** or that **runny-achey flu**.

But it comes with a **sleepy twist**,
A **first-gen antihistamine** on the list.
**Sedation** is common—kids may doze,
Or get **wired** instead (yes, paradox shows!).
It's also used in **emergency care**,
For **anaphylaxis**, as part of the pair—
With **epinephrine** at the head of the team,
Benadryl supports the antihistamine dream.

**Oral**, **IM**, or **IV** route,
Depending on how the symptoms sprout.

**Liquid for kids**, but dose it right—
Too much can cause a scary night.
Side effects? There's quite a few—
**Dry mouth, drowsy, dizzy**, too.
Some get **blurred vision**, or **urinary delay**,
And **constipation** might get in the way.

Overdose is dangerous—watch the signs:
**Hallucinations, seizures**, or strange **declines**.
So **educate parents** to measure with care,
And **avoid double-dosing** unaware.
**Not for infants**, and caution in tots,
Safer meds exist in lots of spots.
No **black box warning**, but still go slow,
And assess **risk vs. benefit** before you go.

Benadryl's classic—nurses know well,
It **calms the itch** and breaks the spell.
But it takes sharp teaching to keep things tight,
So kids get comfort—and sleep at night.

# Diphenhydramine Injection (Benadryl Injection)

*First-Generation Antihistamine*

When **allergies strike** and breathing is tight,
**Benadryl Injection** jumps in to fight.
It's **diphenhydramine**, fast and bold,
To block **histamine** and regain control.
Used for **anaphylaxis**, **severe rash**, or **sting**,
It's part of the rescue, a rapid-acting thing.
Also given for **motion sickness**, or when
**Oral meds fail** or can't begin.

It works on the **H1 histamine crew**,
To stop **swelling**, **itching**, and **wheezing**, too.
But unlike pills, it **acts real fast**,
In **IV** or **IM** when time can't last.
**Side effects** come like they always do—
**Drowsiness**, **dry mouth**, and **blurred vision**, too.
Some kids get **dizzy**, others may shake,
And **low blood pressure** is one to take.

There's risk for **sedation**, or even **confusion**,

And **anticholinergic toxicity** in profusion.

In overdose, you may find

**Tachycardia, seizures**, or **coma in kind**.

So **monitor vitals** closely and well,

And **push it slow** if IV is the spell.

In kids, use weight-based dosing with care,

And **watch the airway**—always be aware.


No **black box warning**, but nurses should know,

It's powerful, fast, and not given slow.

Used best as part of a **rescue plan**,

In allergy crises, it's right-hand man.

**Educate caregivers** what this is for,

Not for mild sniffles or scratches galore.

Benadryl injection is **ER-grade**,

And with **nursing skill**, life-saving aid is made.

# Docusate Sodium (Colace)

*Stool Softener (Emollient Laxative)*

When little ones strain and can't let go,
**Colace** helps the process flow.
**Docusate sodium**, soft and kind,
Eases the stool so it's less confined.
It's not a stimulant, doesn't force,
Just **pulls in water** along the course.
It makes the poop more soft and slick,
So things move out—**gentle and quick**.

Used for **constipation**, mild and slow,
Especially when straining's a big "no-go."
Post-op, post-injury, or after meds,
Colace helps calm those toilet dreads.
**Oral form** is most common in use,
**Liquid or capsule**, with apple juice.
Takes **1 to 3 days** to start its work,
So don't expect a sudden jerk.

Side effects? They're rare, but known:
**Cramping**, **nausea**, or **gas alone**.

If **diarrhea** comes or stool gets thin,
It might be time to check back in.
**Not for long-term use**, be clear—
Or the bowel may forget how to steer.
Encourage **fluids**, **movement**, and **fiber**, too,
So the gut gets help from the whole crew.

There's **no black box**, but still take care,
With infants and toddlers, always beware.
Use only when truly prescribed,
And teach caregivers what's advised.
Colace is gentle, a stool-softening friend,
When nature's stuck and won't descend.
With water, patience, and nursing grace,
It helps little ones go at a gentler pace.

# Electrolyte Oral Solution (Pedialyte)

*Oral Rehydration Solution (ORS)*

When **vomiting** hits or **diarrhea won't quit**,
**Pedialyte** helps kids rally and sit.
It's not just water—it's science inside,
To **replace lost fluids** and **electrolytes** with pride.
**Sodium**, **potassium**, and **glucose, too**,
Balanced just right to **pull fluids through**.
It helps the gut **reabsorb what's lost**,
Without IVs or hospital cost.

Used for **mild to moderate dehydration**,
From stomach bugs or heat sensation.
Given **slowly by mouth**, in careful sips,
To avoid a belly that flips and flips.
Don't mix with juice or water down—
That ruins the ratio that earns its crown.
Offer with spoons or a little cup,
And if they keep it down, just build it up.

**Side effects?** Not really—just do it right,
Too much too fast may cause a fight.
And if the child **can't keep it down**,
Or shows signs of **lethargy or frown**—
**Call the doctor** or head on in,
They may need fluids by IV pin.

No **black box warning**, and **safe when used**,
But it's for **hydration**, not to be abused.
Don't give if there's a full obstruction,
Or if **severe dehydration** needs real suction.
Pedialyte's a **nurse's go-to friend**,
To help the tummy and body mend.
With **patience**, **sips**, and **parent grace**,
It helps little ones get back in the race.

# Epinephrine (EpiPen, Auvi-Q)

*Alpha/Beta Adrenergic Agonist; Emergency Anaphylaxis Med*

When **allergies hit** and breathing's tight,
**EpiPen** comes to save the night.
**Epinephrine**, fast and bold,
A life-saving med that must be told.
It's used in **anaphylaxis**, swift and true,
When swelling, rash, and wheezing brew.
It opens airways, raises the beat,
And helps that **blood pressure** back on its feet.

It works on **alpha and beta receptors**,
To counter the body's allergy tempers.
**Vasoconstriction**, lungs expand,
So oxygen flows just like planned.
It's given **IM**, in the **outer thigh**,
Right through the clothes—don't wait or shy.
Hold for **10 seconds**, then rub the site,
Call **911**, even if they seem right.

**Auto-injectors** like **EpiPen** or **Auvi-Q**,

Make it simple for caregivers to do.
Teach them the signs: **hives**, **swelling**, **wheeze**,
And when to act—with no time to freeze.
**Side effects** may make the heart race fast,
With **tremors**, **sweating**, or nerves that won't last.
But that's expected—it's part of the deal,
When saving a life is the priority real.

No time for slow, no time to wait—
Epi stops the allergic fate.
And after it's given, still go be seen,
For follow-up care and to keep things clean.
There **is a black box**, for **IV use**,
Where dosing errors cause some abuse.
But **auto-injectors** in trained hands,
Are safe and swift—just follow the plans.

Keep one **at school**, one **home**, one **away**,
And **check expiration**—don't let it stay.
Epinephrine's a life-saving friend,
With **nurse education** around every bend.

# Erythromycin Ophthalmic Ointment (Ilotycin)

*Macrolide Antibiotic (Ophthalmic)*

When newborn eyes need **gentle defense**,
**Ilotycin** brings a shield that makes sense.
It's **erythromycin**, smooth and light,
To **prevent infection** and keep vision right.
It's used in babies **just after birth**,
To stop **gonorrhea** or **chlamydia's** worth.
Applied as a **thin strip into each eye**,
Before infections can even try.

It's also used for **conjunctivitis** strain,
When **bacterial pink eye** causes pain.
It stops protein building in the bug's core,
So it **can't reproduce or spread anymore**.
Apply with care—**a ribbon, not a blob**,
Don't touch the tip, just do the job.
**Inner to outer** is how we roll,
Then wipe the excess—gentle is the goal.

Side effects? They're **minimal here**,

Maybe a **blur** or a bit of a tear.

Sometimes the eyes get **red or puffy**,

But allergic response is rare and scruffy.

Teach parents: it may look goopy,

But **don't rinse it out** if it seems too soupy.

Let it stay and do its part,

It's working even if it looks like art.

There's **no black box**, and it's well-tolerated,

For newborn care, it's highly rated.

With **sterile hands** and patient grace,

Ilotycin keeps infection from finding its place.

# Famotidine (Pepcid)

*Histamine-2 Receptor Antagonist (H2 Blocker)*

When **tummies burn** and **acid climbs**,
**Pepcid** helps in quiet times.
It's **famotidine**, cool and mild,
For reflux woes in a gassy child.
It blocks the **H2 histamine gate**,
So **stomach acid** doesn't over-create.
Used for **GERD**, **ulcers**, and tummy pain,
And for **allergic hives** in a different lane.

It's **oral** or **IV**, depending on need,
But **by mouth** is most common for heartburn speed.
Given **with or without food**, that's okay—
But **bedtime doses** work best, they say.
**Side effects** are pretty rare,
But **headache** or **dizzy** might be there.
Some get **constipation**, others get loose,
Or feel a bit **tired**, like a nap's an excuse.

**Long-term use**? Keep labs in check—
It may lower **B12** or leave **labs a wreck**.

Watch for signs of **confusion** or change,
Especially if kidneys are acting strange.
**No black box warning**, but still take care,
Especially if other meds are there.
It may change how some drugs absorb,
So review the list if things feel off-course.

Teach parents to dose it **just as planned**,
And not to double if a dose gets canned.
If symptoms worsen or pain gets strong,
They should follow up—it could be wrong.
Pepcid brings peace to a tummy in fight,
With **nursing support**, it feels just right.
From babies with spit-up to kids who can talk,
It helps little bellies get back on their walk

# Ferrous Sulfate

*Iron Supplement (Oral)*

When **iron is low** and kids feel tired,
With cheeks that pale and moods uninspired,
**Ferrous sulfate** brings strength anew,
To build up blood and energy, too.
It helps make **hemoglobin rise**,
So oxygen flows and focus flies.
Used for **anemia** caused by lack,
It helps get iron stores back on track.

It's given **by mouth**, in **liquid or pill**,
But **tummy troubles** may come still.
**Constipation, nausea**, or **darkened stool**,
Are side effects that follow the rule.
**Give it with juice**, like **vitamin C**,
To boost absorption efficiently.
But never with **milk**—it blocks the flow,
So teach parents what to avoid and know.

Use a **dropper or straw** if liquid form's used,
To avoid stained teeth that can leave them confused.

Brush or rinse right after each dose,

So that little smile stays bright and close.

**Keep it locked up**—one bottle alone

Can cause **iron overdose** on its own.

**Toxic to kids** in high amounts,

So teach safe storage in no uncertain counts.

No **black box warning**, but handle with care,

With **labs to monitor** what's truly there.

Watch **Hgb**, **Hct**, and **ferritin**, too,

To know when to stop or continue through.

It's not a magic fix in a day,

But **daily dosing** clears the way.

With nursing guidance and patient might,

Ferrous sulfate helps blood run bright.

# Fexofenadine (Allegra)

*Second-Generation Antihistamine*

When **sneezing**, **itching**, and **pollen** strike,
**Allegra** helps kids feel just right.
It's **fexofenadine**, calm and clear,
To keep those **seasonal symptoms** in the rear.
It blocks the **H1 histamine line**,
So allergies stop crossing the line.
Great for **hives**, **rhinitis**, and **itchy skin**,
Without the naps that first-gens bring in.

It's a **non-drowsy** med, so kids can play,
And still feel sharp through school all day.
Given **by mouth**, in **tablet or liquid**,
Just once or twice—depends on the ticket.
Take it **with water**, not juice or tea,
Because **fruit juices** block efficacy.
**No food restrictions**, but give it wise—
It works best when symptoms first arise.

Side effects? They're mild and few,
Maybe **headache**, or a **tummy that's blue**.

Rarely, some kids feel **dizzy or tired**,

But usually not enough to feel uninspired.

There's **no black box**, and it's OTC,

But dosing by **weight** is key, you see.

Too much in small kids isn't safe—

So teach caregivers to **measure with grace**.

It's gentle, fast, and widely adored,

For **pollen**, **pets**, or **dust that's stored**.

With fexofenadine in the allergy lane,

Kids can breathe easy and play again.

# Fluoxetine (Prozac)

*Selective Serotonin Reuptake Inhibitor (SSRI)*

When **sadness lingers** or **worries grow**,
**Prozac** helps the healing flow.
It's **fluoxetine**, an SSRI,
To help young minds reach for the sky.
It **blocks reuptake** of serotonin's light,
So more sticks around to feel just right.
Used for **depression**, **OCD**, **anxiety**, too,
And sometimes for **binge eating** breaking through.

It's often the **first SSRI** that's tried,
Because in kids, it's well-studied and wide.
**Given by mouth**, once daily is best,
Usually **in the morning** to avoid sleep unrest.
But don't expect change overnight—
It takes a few **weeks** before things feel right.
And side effects can join at first,
Like **nausea**, **headache**, or **energy burst**.

Some kids feel **jittery**, others feel flat,
So **monitor mood**—and stay aware of that.

**Black box warning**—yes, it's there:
Watch for **suicidal thoughts** with care.
Increased risk in **kids and teens**,
So nurses and parents must read between.
Check in often, track how they feel,
And hold space for feelings that need to heal.

Teach to **take it the same time each day**,
And **don't stop suddenly** or toss it away.
If a dose is missed, don't double or rush,
Just wait for the next—don't cause a crush.
It may cause **weight change**, a **sleepy haze**,
Or **more alertness** in early phase.
But for many, it brings a steadier mind,
And **room to grow** with healing in kind.

# Fluconazole (Diflucan)

*Antifungal (Azole Class)*

When **yeast takes hold** and won't let go,

**Diflucan** helps to stop the show.

**Fluconazole**, an **antifungal ace**,
Targets the root with focused grace.

It **blocks ergosterol** deep inside,

So fungal cells **can't grow or hide**.

Used for **oral thrush, diaper rash**, too,

And **systemic infections** that break right through.

It's given **by mouth**, once daily in dose,

Or **IV** if infections come close.

The **liquid** form works well for tots,

But always **shake it**—no skipping spots.

Side effects? They're usually mild—

A **headache**, or **nausea** in a sensitive child.

But watch the **liver**—it's processed there,

So check those labs with nursing care.

**ALT, AST**, and **bilirubin**,

May rise if the liver isn't in tune.

Rarely, it causes **toxicity signs**,
Like **jaundice**, **dark urine**, or **tired lines**.
It can also cause **QT to extend**,
So check that **EKG** now and then.
And though it's safe when prescribed right,
**Drug interactions** must stay in sight.

It slows down how some **meds break down**,
So double-check with what's already around.
**No black box warning**, but teach the plan—
Complete the course, however it ran.
Fluconazole is small but tough,
One dose for thrush is often enough.
With careful tracking and nursing view,
It helps the body start fresh and new.

# Fluticasone (Flovent)

*Inhaled Corticosteroid (ICS)*

When asthma's a whisper that grows into roar,
**Flovent** helps calm the lungs at the core.
It's **fluticasone**, an inhaled mist,
That keeps **airways open** and **swelling dismissed**.
It's a **corticosteroid**, not a rescue spray,
But a **daily controller** to keep symptoms at bay.
It **reduces inflammation**, clears the path,
So wheezes don't turn into ER wrath.

It's given by **inhaler**, once or twice,
And comes in **diskus**, **HFA**, or **nebulized**.
Not for attacks—that's **albuterol's lane**,
Flovent works in a **long-term game**.
Side effects? **Thrush** may arrive unplanned,
So teach to **rinse the mouth** after each hand.
**Hoarseness**, maybe a **sore throat**, too,
But proper technique will help get through.

**Growth suppression?** A concern that's small,
So we **track their height** and **monitor all**.

Also watch for signs of mood,
Corticosteroids may shift that mood.
No **black box warning**, but still stay sharp,
With **daily weights**, and **lung sound charts**.
And **never stop suddenly**, without a say,
As the body adjusts in its own way.

Teach caregivers this isn't fast,
But over time, it helps lungs last.
With structure, spacing, and nursing grace,
Flovent keeps asthma in a safer place.

# Fluticasone Nasal (Flonase)

*Intranasal Corticosteroid*

When **pollen flies** and noses run,
**Flonase** steps in to get relief begun.
It's **fluticasone**, sprayed up the nose,
To **calm the swelling** and **allergy woes**.
It reduces **inflammation** inside each nare,
So kids can **breathe easy** and sleep with care.
For **seasonal sniffles**, or year-round flare,
It brings relief from the itchy air.

Used for **allergic rhinitis**, both kinds—
**Seasonal** and **chronic**, clearing their minds.
It tackles **sneezing**, **drip**, and **itch**,
But not right away—**it's a slow switch**.
**Once daily dosing** is usually right,
And best if done at the same time each night.
It may take **several days to peak**,
So set expectations and help them speak.

Side effects? They're mostly mild—
A **dry nose** or a **bloody drip** in a child.

Maybe some **headache**, or **burning inside**,
But proper technique can turn that tide.
**Teach to aim away from the septum**, please,
To avoid irritation and nasal unease.
**Prime the spray** if it's brand new,
And **blow the nose first** before they do.

No **black box warning**, but monitor well,
For **slowed growth** in kids—just a little tell.
Track **height and weight** in the growing crew,
Though risk is low, it's what good nurses do.
Flonase helps with each little sneeze,
Turning chaos into calm and breeze.
With steady hands and teaching clear,
Fluticasone keeps those nostrils in gear.

# Fluticasone/Salmeterol (Advair)

*Inhaled Corticosteroid + Long-Acting Beta-2 Agonist (ICS + LABA)*

When asthma's persistent and flares won't fade,
**Advair** brings in a **dual-blade aid**.
It's **fluticasone** for swelling inside,
And **salmeterol** for a bronchodilating ride.
The **steroid calms** the inflamed airway tight,
While **LABA** helps keep breathing light.
It's a **controller med**, not for acute distress,
But to **prevent attacks** and reduce the mess.

Given **twice a day**, one puff at a time,
Through a **Diskus** or **HFA** in rhythmic rhyme.
**Teach to rinse and spit** after each round,
So **thrush** and **hoarseness** won't hang around.
Side effects? They may include:
**Headache**, **tremor**, or a change in mood.
Some feel **restless**, some get sore,
And **tachycardia** can knock on the door.

**LABAs alone** once brought concern,

So now they're paired—**a safer turn**.

There **is a black box warning**, true,

But it's for **monotherapy**, not this combo crew.

Monitor **growth** in kids long-term,

Though the risk is small, we confirm.

Also **watch lung sounds**, and track the score,

If rescue meds are needed more.

Teach families: this is a **daily base**,

To keep flare-ups from showing face.

**Not for sudden wheeze or cough**,

That's albuterol's job to turn it off.

Advair brings balance, control, and flow,

When asthma just won't let go.

With **steady use** and nursing might,

It helps kids breathe and sleep at night.

# Furosemide (Lasix)

*Loop Diuretic*

When **fluid builds up** and lungs feel tight,
**Lasix** helps the body feel light.
It's **furosemide**, strong and fast,
To **pull off fluid** and make swelling pass.
It works in the **loop of Henle's bend**,
Stopping **sodium and water** from reabsorb at the end.
Used for **edema, CHF,** and **renal strain**,
And **hypertension** in a watery chain.

It's given **oral** or by **IV drip**,
But watch that pee—it starts to zip!
**Within an hour**, kids may go,
So plan ahead for that bathroom flow.
But with great power comes some loss—
Like **potassium**, which pays the cost.
Watch for signs of **low K** inside:
**Muscle cramps, weakness,** or **heart that's wide.**

Also check for **low magnesium** and **Na**,
And signs of **dehydration** along the way.

**Daily weights**, and **strict I&Os**,

Let the nurse catch what nobody knows.

It may cause **ototoxicity**,

Especially with **IV given rapidly**.

So **push it slow** and monitor ears,

For **tinnitus** or **hearing that disappears**.

**Photosensitivity** may appear,

So **limit sun** and bring the gear.

Teach parents: **give it early in day**,

So kids aren't peeing the night away.

No **black box warning**, but still proceed,

With **labs**, **BP**, and careful speed.

Lasix works when fluid's too much—

With **nurse precision** and a gentle touch.

# Glycerin Suppositories

*Hyperosmotic Laxative (Rectal)*

When **tummies are full** and poop won't show,
**Glycerin suppositories** help things go.
They work down low, **right where it's stuck**,
Giving the bowels a little luck.
They pull in **water to soften the stool**,
Helping it slide out smooth and cool.
They stimulate gently, right at the end,
So kids can go without meds to send.

Used for **occasional constipation days**,
Especially when oral meds cause delays.
Placed **rectally**, with a gloved-up hand,
And a little lube to help it land.
Works in **15 to 60 minutes**, fast,
So stay nearby—it won't take long to pass!
It's safe for **infants, toddlers**, and **older kids**,
But not for daily poop-schedule bids.

Side effects? Just **mild rectal sting**,
Or a little gas that starts to spring.

But **cramping** or **diarrhea** are rare to see,
And most kids go just fine and pee-free.
**Teach caregivers** to use it wise—
Not too often, and watch the size.
**Infant**, **pediatric**, and **adult forms** vary,
So dosing right is necessary.

There's no **black box**, and it's well-tolerated,
But overuse can get the gut frustrated.
Best used as a **rescue**, not routine,
With fiber, fluids, and veggies between.
For blocked-up bellies and bathroom woes,
Glycerin gives the nudge that flows.
With comfort, care, and timing just right,
It brings relief without a fight.

# Guaifenesin (Mucinex)

*Expectorant*

When coughs are wet and **mucus is thick**,
**Mucinex** helps clear it up quick.
**Guaifenesin** is the name to know,
It helps the **secretions thin and flow**.
It doesn't stop coughs, it makes them clear—
To get the **gunk** out of the chest and near.
Used in **cold**, **bronchitis**, or **sinus blues**,
To break up the junk that the lungs might lose.

It's taken **by mouth**, in **syrup or pill**,
And **extended-release** works longer still.
Push **fluids** with it—it works best that way,
Hydration helps move the mucus away.
Side effects? They're usually light—
Maybe **nausea**, **headache**, or **stomach not right**.
Rarely **rash** or **drowsy fog**,
But mostly it's just clearing the clog.

Teach parents: don't pair it wrong,
With **cough suppressants**, the match is strong—

But sometimes they cancel each other out,
So check the label, and know what it's about.
Not for **kids under two** without the say
Of a **pediatrician**—that's the way.
And if the cough stays more than a week,
It might be time for the doc to peek.

No **black box warning**, and OTC,
But use with care and dosing accuracy.
It doesn't cure, but helps things move—
A mucus-mover in a gentle groove.
So when little lungs are full of goo,
Guaifenesin helps cough it through.
With water, rest, and nursing advice,
It clears the chest and feels quite nice.

# Guanfacine (Intuniv)

*Alpha-2 Adrenergic Agonist (Non-Stimulant ADHD Med)*

When focus is scattered and energy's high,
**Intuniv** helps kids slow down and try.
It's **guanfacine**, a calmer route,
To help with **impulse**, **attention**, and **freak-out**.
It works by **stimulating alpha-2**,
Slowing **norepinephrine** pushing through.
The brain feels less like a buzzing track,
So kids can pause and think right back.

Used for **ADHD**, especially when
**Stimulants fail** or cause mayhem.
It's also used to **lower BP**,
But in peds, it's focus and calm we see.
**Extended-release**, it's taken each day,
Often **at night** to help sleep stay.
It may cause **drowsiness**, **fatigue**, or a chill,
And kids may feel slower—but sometimes still.

Other side effects may include:
**Dry mouth**, **dizzy**, and changes in mood.

And yes—**low blood pressure** is real,
So check **vitals** and note how they feel.
If stopped too fast? That's not wise—
**Rebound hypertension** can quickly rise.
So **taper it slowly**, don't pull away,
Without a plan from the doc in play.

There's **no black box**, but still proceed,
With **monitoring**, patience, and nurse-led speed.
Watch **heart rate**, track **behavior flow**,
And let caregivers know what to watch and show.
Intuniv may not be a cure-all ride,
But it helps kids keep calm from the inside.
With **nursing support** and a tailored plan,
It's one more tool to help them stand.

# Hepatitis B Vaccine

*(Engerix-B, Recombivax HB) Inactivated Recombinant Vaccine*

To **protect the liver** from a viral attack,
The **Hep B vaccine** has our kids' back.
**Engerix-B** or **Recombivax HB**—
It builds immunity silently.
Given **within 24 hours of birth**,
It's one of the **first defenses on Earth**.
Then **1-2 months**, and again at **six**,
A **three-dose series** to seal it quick.

It fights **hepatitis B**, a bloodborne threat,
That scars the liver in ways we regret.
This shot prevents **chronic disease**,
**Cirrhosis**, **cancer**, and more with ease.
It's an **inactivated** recombinant brew,
So it can't cause infection—it just tells the crew.
The immune system trains for a viral fight,
So if it shows up, it knows what's right.

Side effects? They're often mild—

A **sore arm**, a **fussier child**.
Maybe a **low-grade fever**, some redness near,
But serious reactions are **rare to appear**.
**Allergic to yeast**? Then pause this one,
And check with the doc before it's begun.
Otherwise, it's safe and widely used,
And **with breastfeeding, not refused**.

There's **no black box**, but teach the why—
So parents trust, not question or sigh.
This vaccine guards against lifelong pain,
And **early protection** is lifelong gain.
So nurses teach and soothe with care,
While building immunity everywhere.
From day one, it's a gift we give—
To help little livers grow strong and live.

# Hydrochlorothiazide (HCTZ)

*Thiazide Diuretic; Antihypertensive*

When **fluid builds** or **pressure runs high**,
**HCTZ** helps the numbers lie.
**Hydrochlorothiazide**, thiazide class,
Kicks **sodium and water** right out fast.
It works in the **distal tubule's lane**,
To stop salt reabsorption and lessen the strain.
Used for **edema**, **hypertension**, too,
And sometimes for **kidney stones** passing through.

It's taken **orally**, once a day,
Usually **in the morning**—so they're not up halfway.
**Pee increases** and weight might drop,
But we track it all so things don't flop.
**Side effects?** Let's name a few:
**Low potassium**, **low sodium**, too.
Watch for **muscle cramps**, **weakness**, or mood,
And teach them to eat their potassium food.

It can also raise **uric acid** high,
So watch for signs of **gout nearby**.

**Blood sugar** might rise, and **lipids**, too—
So monitor labs as nurses do.
**Photosensitivity** may occur,
So sunscreen talk is part of the cure.
And if a rash or reaction appears,
Stop the med and shift the gears.

No **black box warning**, but we stay aware,
With **electrolyte checks** and thorough care.
**Daily weights, I&Os**, and **BP tracked**,
Keep side effects safely stacked.
So when fluids rise or pressure won't yield,
HCTZ takes the field.
With nurse support and education strong,
This med helps kids feel right where they belong.

# Hydrocortisone Cream (Cortizone)

*Topical Corticosteroid (Low Potency)*

When **skin flares up** with a rash or bite,
**Cortizone cream** helps make it right.
**Hydrocortisone**, smooth and mild,
Brings comfort fast to an itchy child.
It calms the **inflammation, redness, and swell**,
And helps where **eczema** or **bug bites** dwell.
From **contact rashes** to **diaper heat**,
It soothes the spots from head to feet.

It's a **low-strength steroid**, safe and light,
But still must be **used just right**.
Apply a **thin layer**, not too thick,
And never **under dressings** unless it's quick.
**Twice a day** is usually enough,
And more than a **week** can get rough.
Too much use can thin the skin,
So limit the time it's rubbed in.

**Not for open wounds or eyes**, oh no—
And not inside where creams don't go.

If the rash gets worse or starts to spread,
That's when it's time to see the ped.
Side effects? They're rare and few,
But **burning** or **itching** might peek through.
And overuse in the diaper zone,
Could lead to **thinner skin tone**.

No **black box warning**, but teach with care—
That **less is more** when applying there.
And **wash your hands** when the cream is through,
So steroids don't go where they're not due.
For itchy kids with bumps and woes,
Hydrocortisone keeps calm in those.
With nurse direction and parent grace,
It soothes the skin and heals the space.

# Hydroxyzine (Atarax, Vistaril)

*First-Generation Antihistamine; Anxiolytic; Sedative*

When **itching won't stop** or **nerves run high**,
**Hydroxyzine** helps those symptoms fly.
Known as **Atarax** or **Vistaril**,
It calms the skin—and the mind—at will.
It's an **H1 blocker**, first-gen class,
That also helps **anxious feelings** pass.
Used for **hives, eczema**, or **sleepless nights**,
And even for **pre-op calming** frights.

It's taken **by mouth**, or sometimes **IM**,
Depending on what you're treating then.
**Liquid or tablet**, it's easy to give,
And helps little ones rest and live.
Side effects? Yes, there are a few:
**Drowsiness, dry mouth**, and **foggy view**.
Some kids get **dizzy**, a **bit withdrawn**,
But most effects are mild and gone.

**CNS depression** can be real,
So watch for **sedation** and how they feel.

It shouldn't mix with other meds

That make them sleepy or dull their heads.

**No black box warning**, but still advise:

Use caution in **seizure-prone** or sleepy eyes.

**QT prolongation** is rare but true—

So watch the EKG if risk runs through.

Teach parents: it's not for daily sneeze,

But more for **itching**, **nerves**, or **ease**.

Take it **as needed** or **scheduled tight**,

And give at **bedtime** if it brings night-light.

Hydroxyzine is versatile and sweet,

Helping kids stay calm and neat.

With **nurse support** and the right dose shared,

It brings relief when they're itchy or scared.

# Ibuprofen (Advil, Motrin)

*Nonsteroidal Anti-Inflammatory Drug (NSAID)*

When **fevers rise** or **tummies ache**,
**Ibuprofen** gives a gentle break.
Known as **Advil** or **Motrin** on the shelf,
It helps kids **feel more like themselves**.
It's an **NSAID**, reducing **fever and pain**,
And calming down **inflammatory strain**.
From **teething**, **sore throat**, or a **sprained little knee**,
It brings relief quite reliably.

It blocks the **COX enzyme's** usual track,
So **prostaglandins** don't fight back.
That means less swelling, less heat, less fuss,
And more time to heal—without much muss.
Give it **by mouth**, with food if you can,
To **protect the stomach** as part of the plan.
Dosing's based on **weight**, not just age—
So check that chart before turning the page.

It lasts around **6 to 8 hours**, long,
But **don't exceed** the daily song.

Too much can hurt the **kidneys inside**,

So space those doses and let time guide.

Side effects? **Tummy upset**, perhaps,

Or **nausea, gas**, or **occasional lapse**

In appetite. And if taken too deep,

It may cause **GI bleeding** or a **kidney beep**.

**No black box for kids** at play,

But **long-term use** should be guided each day.

Avoid it in **dehydration zones**,

Or when viral fevers bring unknown tones.

Teach caregivers how to measure it right,

Not just a kitchen spoon at night.

And don't pair with other NSAIDs in tow—

**Acetaminophen** is the safer duo.

Ibuprofen's trusted, strong, and mild,

A comfort tool for any child.

With **nursing guidance** and dosing done true,

It helps small bodies feel good as new.

# Influenza Vaccine (Fluzone – Injection, FluMist – Nasal Spray)

*Inactivated or Live Attenuated Vaccine*

When **flu season hits** and germs fill the air,
The **flu shot** steps in to help kids prepare.
Whether **Fluzone** (a shot) or **FluMist** (a spray),
Both guard the body in a powerful way.
The **injectable version** is tried and true—
It's **inactivated**, safe to do.
It's given **IM**, in the leg or the arm,
To protect from **fever**, **fatigue**, and harm.

**FluMist** is sprayed in the nose with care,
A **live attenuated** option there.
No needle in sight, just sniff and done—
But it's **not for all kids**, even if fun.
FluMist is **only for healthy kids**,
**Age 2 and up**—no asthma bids.
No use if **immunocompromised** inside,
Or with **aspirin therapy** alongside.

Flu shots are safe for **6 months and older**,

Protecting kids as weather gets colder.

Side effects? Just a **sore spot** or two,

A **mild fever**, or a **runny nose** might come through.

But the flu itself? It can be rough—

With **body aches**, **coughing**, and breathing tough.

So we vaccinate each year on time,

As the flu strains shift and climb.

No **black box warning**, but teach the facts—

That **some protection** is better than cracks.

It may not stop every strain in the race,

But it **lowers the risk** of a hospital place.

Teach families: even if kids still get sick,

They bounce back faster, and symptoms aren't thick.

With **nurse support** and education clear,

We help fight the flu each and every year.

# Insulin (Humulin, Novolog, Lantus)

*Hormone Replacement – Blood Glucose Regulator*

When **blood sugar climbs** and won't come down,
**Insulin** steps in to smooth the crown.
It's the key for kids with **type 1** in play,
And sometimes for **type 2** along the way.
**Humulin** comes in **Regular** and **NPH**,
One's **short-acting**, the other—**mid-stretch**.
**Novolog** is **rapid**, works real fast,
Great before meals—but it won't last.

Then there's **Lantus, long and slow**,
It lasts all day with a **steady flow**.
**Basal insulin**, quiet and deep,
Keeps sugar steady—even in sleep.
Each type has its time and pace,
So **know your insulin**, don't misplace.
They **lower glucose**, help cells take it in,
Fueling muscles and organs within.

**Side effects?** The main one's clear—
**Hypoglycemia**, creeping near.

Shakiness, sweat, and feeling low,

Kids may cry or not even know.

So **check blood sugar** before and after,

And keep some juice nearby for faster.

Too much insulin, food too late,

Can send them into a hypoglycemic state.

**Rotate sites** if given by shot,

**Thighs, arms, abdomen**—change the spot.

**Don't mix Lantus** with other meds,

And store all insulin in cool homesteads.

**Teach caregivers** to track the signs,

Of highs and lows, and dosing lines.

Use **carb counting, activity logs**,

And always carry supplies in bags or jogs.

No **black box warning**, but still go slow,

And educate so they **really know**.

Insulin saves and gives control,

With **nursing care**, kids reach their goal.

# Lactulose (Generlac)

*Osmotic Laxative; Ammonia Reducer*

When **poop is stuck** or **ammonia's high**,
**Lactulose** helps things pass right by.
It's sweet and sticky, thick and slow,
But helps the **gut and bowels flow**.
It draws in **water to soften the stool**,
And keeps things moving—that's the rule.
Used in **constipation**, stubborn and tough,
And for **hepatic encephalopathy stuff**.

In liver disease, it clears the track,
By pulling **ammonia** down and back.
Traps it in the gut, so it won't roam—
And sends it out before it finds home.
**Given by mouth**, or **rectally placed**,
It works within hours—sometimes in haste.
**Titrate the dose** so they poop just right,
Not too loose, and not all night.

Side effects? Let's name a few:
**Gas**, **bloating**, and **cramps** may come through.

**Diarrhea** means the dose is high,

Or they're dehydrated—keep an eye.

**Electrolyte shifts** can tag along,

So check their labs if it lasts too long.

**Sodium low** or **potassium out**,

Are things we watch and care about.

There's no **black box**, but we still guide,

With nursing checks right by their side.

Teach parents: the taste is sweet,

But **mix with juice** to make it neat.

Lactulose helps the system reset,

For liver relief or bathroom bet.

With **hydration**, care, and nurse review,

It keeps things moving like they're meant to do.

# Lamotrigine (Lamictal)

*Anticonvulsant; Mood Stabilizer*

When **seizures flash** or **moods swing wide**,
**Lamotrigine** helps stabilize the ride.
It calms the brain's electric tide,
So waves of storm can gently subside.
Used for **epilepsy**, from small to grand,
And **bipolar disorder**, when moods expand.
It helps prevent the crashing low,
And slows the spikes that start to grow.

It **blocks sodium channels** in the brain,
To calm the nerves and reduce the strain.
Given **by mouth**, it starts out slow,
With careful titration as levels grow.
Why so slow? Because of a risk—
**Stevens-Johnson syndrome**—rare, but brisk.
A **rash** can mean it's time to stop,
And nurses must teach what signs should pop.

**Dizziness**, **nausea**, and **blurry view**,
**Sleepiness** may also come through.

Mood may shift—or calm instead,
So **watch behavior** and what's being said.
Used in **teens and children**, too,
But **dosing by weight** is what we do.
Check for **interactions** in the med list pile—
Valproate, for one, can change its style.

No **black box warning**, but the rash alert
Makes **early teaching** a nursing perk.
Tell families: report signs right away,
Don't wait for the symptoms to worsen or stay.
Lamotrigine brings balance and calm,
A steady hand, a mental balm.
With nurses guiding dose and plan,
It helps young brains the best it can.

# Levalbuterol (Xopenex)

*Short-Acting Beta-2 Adrenergic Agonist (SABA)*

When **wheezing starts** and lungs feel tight,
**Xopenex** helps the airways fight.
It's **levalbuterol**, fast and clean,
A **rescue inhaler** from the beta-2 team.
It relaxes muscles deep in the chest,
So kids can breathe and catch their rest.
Used for **asthma** or **bronchospasm flare**,
It opens the lungs and clears the air.

Compared to albuterol, it may bring less,
Of the **shaky hands** and **heart-pounding stress**.
It's **more selective**, a purer start,
Still acting fast—but gentler on the heart.
Given by **inhaler** or **nebulized mist**,
Every **4 to 6 hours**, when needed on the list.
Always **listen to lungs** before and after,
And track how well they breathe with laughter.

**Side effects** can still include:
**Tachycardia, tremors**, or **mood subdued**.

**Nausea, nervousness, dizzy spells,**
And rarely, chest pain that rings alarm bells.
Teach parents: it's not for daily control,
That's what **inhaled steroids** are for, on the whole.
This is for **rescue**, when symptoms peak—
To stop the wheeze and help them speak.

No **black box warning**, but caution still,
Especially with **cardiac history or chill**.
Track response, teach the cues,
So families know when and how to use.
Levalbuterol works fast and true,
With nurse support, it's safer too.
A breath of relief in a pocket-sized tool,
Keeping lungs open, calm, and cool.

# Levetiracetam (Keppra)

*Anticonvulsant*

When **seizures strike** and won't behave,
**Keppra** steps in the brain to save.
It's **levetiracetam**, steady and strong,
To help stop seizures from lasting too long.
Used for **partial**, **tonic-clonic**, and more,
In kids as young as one month or before.
It doesn't slow sodium like others do,
But binds to brain proteins to help push through.

It's taken **by mouth** or **IV line**,
With **twice-a-day dosing**, most of the time.
No need for titration at the start,
But **adjust by weight**—that's the key part.
**Side effects** may include:
**Drowsiness**, **fatigue**, or **mood that's skewed**.
**Irritability** is known in some,
So monitor mood as seizures come.

**Behavioral shifts**—aggression, tears,
May happen in kids, especially with fears.

Also watch for **dizzy** or **coordination delay**,
Especially early in the treatment play.
No **black box warning**, but watch the signs,
Of **suicidal thoughts** in pediatric minds.
And never stop it all at once—
**Withdrawal seizures** pack a punch.

It doesn't play rough with other meds,
But still review the list that's read.
**Liver-safe**, and no blood draws often,
A med that many docs choose soften'.
Keppra's calm, but nurse-aware,
With **teaching**, **tracking**, and gentle care.
With families, plans, and seizure logs,
It helps bring peace through mental fogs.

# Levothyroxine (Synthroid)

*Thyroid Hormone Replacement*

When a **tiny thyroid** isn't enough,
**Synthroid** steps in with powerful stuff.
**Levothyroxine**, a daily aid,
Keeps **metabolism properly laid**.
Used in **hypothyroidism**, young or old,
It helps the **heart**, **growth**, and **mind unfold**.
From **congenital cases** caught at birth,
To **Hashimoto's** or slower worth.

It's a **synthetic T4** hormone ride,
Converted to T3 once inside.
It works best when taken alone,
On an **empty stomach**, in the morning zone.
**Side effects** from too much may show:
**Sweating**, **weight loss**, or **heart that goes go-go**.
Too little? Then signs may appear:
**Fatigue**, **cold hands**, or **thinking unclear**.
**Dosing is delicate**, weight-based, and tight,

With **frequent labs** to get it right.

**TSH**, **T4**, and growth we track,

To make sure hormone levels come back.

No **black box warning**, but dose with care—

Too much can tip the cardiac flair.

And teach parents not to skip or change,

Unless the doctor makes the range.

Tablets, **crushed** for infants small,

Can mix with water—not food at all.

**Soy**, **iron**, and **calcium** can interfere,

So give them far from dosing—keep it clear.

Levothyroxine keeps bodies in line,

So kids can grow and feel just fine.

With nurse support and timing true,

It keeps the body steady and new.

# Lisdexamfetamine (Vyvanse)

*Central Nervous System Stimulant; ADHD Med*

When **focus is hard** and the mind's on spin,
**Vyvanse** helps bring attention in.
It's **lisdexamfetamine**, long and lean,
A **prodrug stimulant**—clean and keen.
Used for **ADHD** in kids and teens,
To help with **impulse**, **focus**, and **daily routines**.
Also used for **binge eating** in older youth,
It sharpens the mind with lasting truth.

It converts to **dextroamphetamine** inside,
Where liver and enzymes gently guide.
That means **smoother release**—less crash at the end,
With **12-hour action** to help them attend.
Given **by mouth**, early in day,
So sleep won't get in the stimulant's way.
**Capsules or chewables**, both are here,
But **don't crush or snort**—make that clear.

**Side effects** may still appear:
**Decreased appetite**, **dry mouth**, or **fear**,

**Irritability**, **insomnia**, or mood that swings,
Even **tics** or emotional things.
It may raise **heart rate** or **blood pressure**, too,
So **vitals and growth** checks are what we do.
And screen for **misuse**, especially in teens—
This med's controlled, if you know what that means.

There **is a black box warning** to state:
**Abuse and dependency**—don't medicate late.
**Taper it off** if it's time to stop,
To avoid withdrawal or energy drop.
Teach caregivers all the signs,
Track **meals**, **mood**, and dosing times.
Vyvanse brings focus and calm in stride,
With **nurse support** right by their side.

# Loperamide (Imodium)

*Antidiarrheal; Opioid-Receptor Agonist (Peripherally Acting)*

When **tummies rumble** and **stools won't stop**,
**Imodium** helps slow the drop.
**Loperamide** works to calm the gut,
And firm up stools when things go... abrupt.
It binds to **opioid receptors** down low,
To **slow peristalsis** and make things flow.
Used for **acute diarrhea**, sometimes **chronic**,
But not for bugs that are viral or colonic.

It **doesn't cross the blood-brain line**,
So it won't cause highs—but slows just fine.
It helps reduce **frequency, cramps**, and fear,
When dehydration starts to near.
**Given by mouth**, in **liquid or chew**,
But **not approved in young infants** too.
Generally **over age 2 with caution**,
And under **close pediatrician supervision**.

**Side effects** are mostly mild:
**Bloating, nausea**, or a sleepy child.

But too much can **stop things cold**,

Causing **constipation** or symptoms bold.

If there's **blood in the stool**, or **fever** present,

Imodium use is **not** what's meant.

It can **trap infections** inside the gut,

Which could lead to something worse... and shut.

There's **no black box**, but don't be lax—

Improper use can cause setbacks.

**Torsades**, **ileus**, or CNS signs

Occur when **abused**, especially in high lines.

Teach parents to **push fluids**, too,

And **monitor diapers** for output and hue.

Imodium calms when used with care,

But **nursing guidance** must be there.

# Loratadine (Claritin)

*Second-Generation Antihistamine*

When **pollen floats** and **noses sneeze**,
**Claritin** helps bring kids some ease.
**Loratadine** works without the yawn,
So they can play from dusk till dawn.
It blocks the **H1 histamine way**,
To keep **itching**, **hives**, and **drip** at bay.
Used for **seasonal allergies** and more,
Like **chronic urticaria** itching sore.

It's **non-drowsy**, which is great for school,
And **once a day** is the usual rule.
**Liquid**, **chewable**, or **tablet form**,
It keeps them clear through allergy storm.
**Side effects** are light and rare:
Maybe **headache** or a **tummy flare**.
But it's well-tolerated in most who try,
With **no sedation** to make them lie.

No **black box warning**, no major scare,
Just proper dosing and nurse-led care.

Avoid in kids under **two years old**,

Unless the provider gives the gold.

Teach families to **read OTC labels right**,

To avoid **accidental double-dose fright**.

It's often mixed in combo meds,

So check each bottle before it's fed.

Loratadine keeps the sneezes back,

Without the **fog** or **energy lack**.

A gentle friend through allergy season,

With **nurse guidance** and a clear-breath reason.

# MMR Vaccine (M-M-R II)

*Live Attenuated Vaccine – Measles, Mumps, Rubella*

To guard against **three viral foes**,
The **MMR vaccine** clearly knows.
**M-M-R II** is the name you'll see,
Protecting kids from **disease x3**.
**Measles** brings rash, with cough and red eyes,
It spreads through air and multiplies.
**Mumps** swells cheeks and glands so sore,
While **Rubella** can harm unborns and more.

This vaccine is **live**, but **weakened down**,
To build strong shields without the crown.
Given at **12–15 months**, then again at **four**,
Two doses help immunity soar.
It's **subcutaneous**, in the thigh or arm,
With tiny discomfort—but **huge charm**.
Side effects? Usually **mild and neat**:
A **low fever**, or **rash**, or **swelling at feet**.

Sometimes a **febrile seizure** may appear,
But it's rare—and nurses stay near.

**Joint pain** can happen in older youth,

But symptoms pass—and that's the truth.

**Not for the immunocompromised** crowd,

Or **pregnant teens** (live rules aren't allowed).

If allergic to **gelatin** or **neomycin trace**,

Then skip this shot, or test in place.

**No black box warning**, but nurse must teach,

That **measles outbreaks** are still in reach.

So every dose protects us all—

From school to plane to shopping mall.

Teach parents it's **not linked to fear**,

Autism myths have been made clear.

MMR is safe and strong and wise—

And helps our kids immunize.

# Mebendazole (Emverm)

*Anthelmintic (Anti-Worm Medication)*

When **worms creep in** and cause distress,
**Emverm** helps clean up the mess.
**Mebendazole** is what we give,
To help those **parasites cease to live**.
It's used for **pinworms**, **roundworms**, and more,
Creepy-crawly guests we all abhor.
It **blocks glucose uptake** in the worm,
So they **starve and die**—no chance to squirm.

Given **by mouth**, it's often one dose,
But sometimes a **repeat** keeps things close.
Chewable tablets, simple and sweet,
Make deworming easier to complete.
Side effects? They're usually few:
Maybe **cramps**, **gas**, or **loose stool** too.
**Rare rash**, **dizzy**, or **itchy skin**,
But most kids tolerate it well within.

Teach parents it's **best with food**,
And if **pinworms** spread in siblinghood—

Treat the whole **household all the same**,
To stop the cycle and end the game.
Clean **clothes**, **bedding**, and **fingers**, too,
Because those eggs can stick like glue.
Trim nails short, wash hands right,
And avoid reinfection night after night.

No **black box warning**, but still take care,
Especially in **long-term use** that's rare.
Check for **pregnancy**—don't medicate
Until the provider clears the gate.
Mebendazole clears the parasite fuss,
With **nursing guidance**, and trust in us.
One tiny tablet, and life feels right—
No more wiggles in bed at night.

# Melatonin

*Sleep Aid; Hormone Supplement*

When **bedtime battles** start to rise,
And tired kids rub sleepy eyes,
Some parents turn to **melatonin's glow**,
To help their little ones rest and slow.
It's a **natural hormone**, made at night,
By the **pineal gland** when it dims the light.
It helps the body **know when to sleep**,
So minds can calm and dreams run deep.

Used for **insomnia, ADHD sleep delay**,
**Autism**, or **jet lag** on travel day.
It doesn't knock out like meds you've known—
It's more a **gentle nudge** toward sleep zone.
Given **by mouth**, in **liquid or chew**,
**30 minutes before bed** will usually do.
**Start with low doses**, slow and light—
Sometimes too much can backfire at night.

**Side effects?** They're mostly few:
**Morning grogginess**, or a mood that's blue.

Some kids may get vivid dreams,
Or feel off-track with melatonin schemes.
It's not FDA-approved for youth,
But widely used—and that's the truth.
So nurses teach with care and voice,
To help parents make an informed choice.

**No black box warning**, but guidance is key,
It's not for every family's sleep decree.
Long-term use? That's still debated,
So check with a doc before it's created.
Teach healthy habits:
▫ **Same bedtime**,
 **Screens down**,
▫ **Dim the lights**,
 **Wind-down time**.

Melatonin may help the sleep fight end,
But it works best with **routine as its friend**.
With **nurse support**, and structure tight,
Kids find their rhythm and sleep at night.

# Methotrexate

*Antimetabolite; Immunosuppressant; Disease-Modifying Antirheumatic Drug (DMARD)*

When the **immune system fights too strong**,

**Methotrexate** helps calm what's wrong.

It slows down cells that grow too fast,

To **ease inflammation** and **make comfort last**.

Used for **juvenile arthritis pain**,

Or in **leukemia** to stop cell gain.

Also for **lupus**, **psoriasis**, too—

It tells the body what *not* to do.

It's a **folic acid blocker**, deep,

That slows DNA so cells won't leap.

Given **by mouth**, **IM**, or **subQ** style,

Once a week, with labs on file.

**Side effects** range mild to bold:

**Nausea**, **mouth sores**, or a **tummy cold**.

Fatigue, low counts, or **hair that sheds**,

And **liver toxicity** must be kept in our heads.

So nurses check with labs in hand—

**CBC**, **LFTs**, and all that's planned.
Watch for signs of **infection risk**,
And teach families not to dismiss.
It has a **black box warning**, too—
For **organ damage** and **immune issues** that brew.
Never use in **pregnancy stage**,
It's **teratogenic** across the page.

Pair with **folic acid** day by day,
To help side effects stay away.
Teach to take it **same day each week**,
And **call the doc** if things feel weak.
Avoid **NSAIDs**, or alcohol fun,
To keep the liver from coming undone.
With nurse support, labs, and care,
Methotrexate works when plans are fair.

# Methylphenidate (Ritalin, Concerta, Metadate)

*Central Nervous System Stimulant; ADHD Medication*

When **focus is fleeting** and thoughts run fast,
**Methylphenidate** helps attention last.
Known as **Ritalin**, **Concerta**, or **Metadate**,
It helps kids sit still, think clear, and regulate.
It boosts **dopamine** and **norepinephrine flow**,
So **attention**, **impulse**, and **focus** grow.
Used for **ADHD** throughout the day,
It helps the brain find a better way.

**Short-acting**, **long**, or **extended-release**,
Dosed in the morning to work in peace.
**Tablets**, **capsules**, or **liquid to take**,
Each version tailored for how long it'll wake.
Side effects? There's quite a few:
**Decreased appetite**, **trouble sleeping**, too.
**Tics**, **irritability**, or a **racing heart**,
So monitor mood and how they start.

Check **height and weight**—they might slow,
And **BP**, **HR** with each dose they go.
May cause **dry mouth**, **headache**, or **nausea**, mild—
But often calms an overwhelmed child.
There **is a black box warning** in place,
For **abuse potential** and **misuse case**.
It's a **controlled substance**, locked up tight,
So teach families to store it right.

Don't stop it suddenly—**taper with care**,
And avoid **late doses** or sleep's unfair.
Best given **early**, with food or none,
To avoid the crash when day is done.
With **nursing checks**, routine, and plan,
This med can help like few things can.
It sharpens minds and slows the race,
So kids can thrive in every space.

# Metronidazole (Flagyl)

*Antibiotic; Antiprotozoal*

When **germs go low** in the gut or below,
**Flagyl** is the one that steals the show.
**Metronidazole**, a tough little star,
Fights **anaerobes** that don't travel far.
Used for **C. diff**, **trich**, and **bacterial vaginosis**,
Or **giardia bugs** causing GI neurosis.
Also for **dental**, **abdominal**, or **pelvic infection**,
It's the go-to for targeted gut protection.

It **disrupts DNA** in cells that grow,
So bacteria die and symptoms go.
**Given by mouth**, **IV**, or **topical cream**,
It works through the bloodstream like a dream.
Side effects? You might see:
**Nausea**, **metallic taste**, **GI plea**.
Sometimes **headache**, **dark urine**, too—
All normal things it can put you through.

But there's a warning loud and bold:
**No alcohol**—not young, not old.

It can cause a **disulfiram-like crash**,

With **vomiting**, **flushing**, and a whole-body flash.

**Dosing by weight** in kids, of course,

And **give with food** if it's a rough course.

Finish the **full prescription round**,

Even if symptoms don't stick around.

There's **no black box**, but caution is key—

Especially with **long-term neurotoxicity**.

Watch for **seizures**, **numbness**, or gait that's off,

And call the provider at the very first cough.

Flagyl works where oxygen's rare,

In **deep infections**, it gets in there.

With **nurse-led care** and good instruction,

It clears the path to smooth gut function.

# Midazolam (Versed)

*Benzodiazepine; Sedative; Anticonvulsant*

When **panic spikes** or **seizures flare**,
**Versed** brings calm with nursing care.
**Midazolam** is smooth and fast,
For moments when **urgency's moving past**.
It's a **benzo**, working deep in the brain,
Boosting **GABA** to ease the strain.
Used for **procedural sedation** and **status control**,
It helps restless minds regain control.

**Intranasal**, **IM**, or **IV** stream,
It kicks in fast like a steady dream.
In emergencies, it's a seizure stop,
When **Diastat** isn't the one on top.
Side effects? They're part of the deal:
**Respiratory depression** is very real.
Also **hypotension**, **bradycardia**, and more—
So monitor closely on the hospital floor.

**Continuous monitoring** is a must,
With oxygen, suction, and nursing trust.

And always have **flumazenil** near,

In case reversal is needed here.

**Black box warning**—yes, it's true:

**Respiratory risk** and **sedation, too**.

Especially when mixed with other CNS meds,

It can slow down breathing or sleepy heads.

Used carefully, it calms the storm,

In anxious hearts or brains not warm.

With **tight nurse watch** and patient grace,

Versed brings stillness to a racing place.

# Mometasone Nasal (Nasonex)

*Intranasal Corticosteroid*

When **allergy season** clogs the nose,
**Nasonex** helps the swelling close.
**Mometasone**, sprayed once a day,
Keeps **itchy sneezes** and **drip** away.
It's a **steroid** that works right where it's sprayed,
To stop **inflammation** before it's displayed.
Great for **rhinitis**, both **seasonal** and **chronic**,
It makes stuffy days less iconic.

It won't bring sleep or wired moods,
Like antihistamines often intrude.
But it **takes a few days** before relief is felt,
So teach to stick with it—don't melt.
Side effects? They're usually mild:
A **nosebleed**, or **burning** in a sensitive child.
Sometimes **headache**, or a dry nose sting,
But overall, it's a gentle thing.

Teach kids to **blow before they spray**,
And **aim away from the septum** each day.

**Rinse the nozzle**, and store it clean,

So the next dose stays fresh and keen.

No **black box warning**, but nurses should track

Signs of **slowed growth** in kids, way back.

Though rare, it's wise to monitor height,

And review progress at each new light.

Mometasone clears the nasal mess,

With **daily use and nurse finesse**.

Helping kids breathe through allergy strife,

So they can smile and get on with life.

# Montelukast (Singulair)

*Leukotriene Receptor Antagonist (LTRA)*

When **asthma flares** or **allergies stay**,
**Singulair** helps keep symptoms at bay.
**Montelukast** blocks the path so tight,
Where **leukotrienes** fuel the swelling fight.
Used for **chronic asthma**, not rescue style,
And for **seasonal sniffles** that last a while.
Also used to **prevent exercise wheeze**,
It helps lungs open and symptoms ease.

**Given by mouth**, once daily at night,
So breathing stays smooth through morning light.
Comes in **chewables**, **granules**, or pill,
Depending on age and swallow skill.
Side effects? Most do fine,
But some may show a mood decline.
**Nightmares**, **agitation**, **anxious minds**,
**Depression**, or thoughts of the darkest kinds.

So **nurses teach** and **families track**,
Any **behavioral changes** that circle back.

Though rare, there's now a **boxed warning** here,
For **neuropsychiatric effects** that appear.
It's **not a steroid**, and won't replace,
Your **daily inhaler** in asthma's case.
It's **add-on therapy**, not stand-alone,
But helpful when triggers are fully known.

Avoid giving with **Phenobarb** or **Rifampin**,
Those speed its clearance—less stays within.
And teach to stick to the **same time each day**,
So the med can work in a steady way.
Montelukast helps **lungs feel free**,
When used with care and consistency.
With nurse support and questions clear,
Singulair can bring easier air.

# Multivitamin with Iron (Poly-Vi-Sol)

*Pediatric Multivitamin Supplement with Iron*

When little ones grow and iron runs low,
**Poly-Vi-Sol** helps the nutrients flow.
A **multivitamin with iron inside**,
To help support growth on the daily ride.
Used for **infants and toddlers** alike,
When **diet is limited** or iron's on strike.
It fills in gaps from veggies or meat,
To help small bodies feel complete.

**Iron builds blood**, while **vitamins boost**
Bones, brains, and muscles on the loose.
Essential for kids who were born a bit small,
Or need a supplement to give it their all.
**Given by dropper**, it's sticky and sweet,
But it can stain **teeth**—so rinse or eat.
**Mix with juice or food** to help it go down,
And **never give lying flat**—help them sit or crown.

Side effects? Mostly **tummy woes**,
Like **constipation** or **blackened poos**.

Too much iron is dangerous still—

So **lock the bottle** to avoid any spill.

**Iron overdose** is real and fast,

So teach parents that safety must last.

**One dose a day** is all they need,

Measured with care—not done by speed.

No **black box warning**, but nurse eyes stay

On growth, diet, and labs along the way.

With **daily dosing**, the job is done,

Helping little bodies rise and run.

# Mupirocin (Bactroban)

*Topical Antibiotic*

When **cuts get red** or **skin gets sore**,
**Bactroban** helps the bugs no more.
**Mupirocin** fights the local flair,
Stopping **bacterial growth** right there.
Used for **impetigo**, **scrapes**, and small wounds,
It clears the skin in just a few moons.
Also used in **MRSA nose care**,
But most often it's for **topical repair**.

It stops **protein synthesis** on the spot,
So bacteria die and wounds do not rot.
Applied **three times daily** in a thin spread,
Just enough to turn infection on its head.
**Side effects?** They're rare and light—
**Stinging**, **burning**, or **rash in sight**.
If skin worsens or swelling grows,
It's time to stop and let the doc know.

Teach to use it **only as prescribed**,
Not for **fungal rashes** or over-applied.

Don't share tubes or rub it wide—

Just **small, clean spots**, and seal with pride.

No **black box warning**, and it's well-tolerated,

But long-term use? Not advocated.

Mupirocin clears what's trying to stay,

And **heals the skin** the nursing way.

# Nitrofurantoin (Macrobid, Macrodantin)

*Urinary Tract Antibiotic*

When **UTIs strike** and cause a fuss,
**Macrobid** steps in to fight with us.
**Nitrofurantoin**, small but strong,
Targets **bladder bugs** that don't belong.
It **damages bacterial DNA**,
So infection fades and clears the way.
Used for **lower UTIs**, not kidneys or more—
It's not for infections that rise and soar.

**Macrobid** is a **longer-release** form,
**Macrodantin**—**shorter**, taken more norm.
Given **by mouth**, with **food on the plate**,
To help absorption and feel great.
Side effects? Let's name a few:
**Nausea, headache,** or **urine that's blue**
(Yellow or brown—that's sometimes seen,
It's **harmless**, though it may look unclean).

But here's the warning nurses know:
In **infants under 1 month**, it's a no-go.
It risks **hemolytic anemia** fast,
So check age and weight before you cast.
And if used long, watch for signs
Of **lung trouble** or **nerve tingling lines**.
Rare risks include **pulmonary reaction**,
So teach to report any cough in action.

No **black box warning**, but still take care,
In **renal impairment**, it's not quite fair.
Avoid if **creatinine's high**,
So dose adjustments might apply.
Teach families to **complete the med**,
Even when symptoms start to shed.
Hydrate well and take on time—
So those UTI bugs can't re-climb.

Nitrofurantoin clears the way,
When bladder bugs try to overstay.
With nursing care and timing true,
It helps kids feel like **themselves anew**.

# Nystatin (Mycostatin)
*Antifungal (Polyene Class)*

When **yeast takes hold** in mouth or skin,
**Mycostatin** helps healing begin.
**Nystatin** targets the fungal spread,
So **candida clears** and comfort's ahead.
Used for **oral thrush**, so common and white,
Or **diaper rash** that doesn't feel right.
It binds to **ergosterol** in the yeast cell wall,
Causing it to **leak** and eventually fall.

**Oral suspension**—swish or paint,
For infants too young to spit or faint.
Apply **to cheeks, tongue**, and **gums** with care,
And remind them not to swallow air.
For **skin**, use **cream** in a thin, smooth way,
**Twice a day** is the usual play.
Keep the area **clean and dry**,
And **cotton clothes** help moisture fly.

**Side effects?** Just mild, if any—
Like **skin irritation**, but not too many.

**Bitter taste** or a **tummy flare**,
But allergic reactions are truly rare.
**No black box warning**, no deep alarm,
But it still should be **used with calm**.
Not for **systemic infections** wide—
This one works on the **outside** side.

Teach caregivers to **finish the round**,
Even if symptoms can't be found.
And never mix with diaper cream foes,
Unless the provider clearly knows.
Nystatin works when yeast won't quit,
With **nurse support** and just the right kit.
It brings back comfort, smiles, and ease—
So little ones heal and parents breathe.

# Ofloxacin Otic (Floxin Otic)

When **ears are sore** and **drainage flows**,
**Floxin Otic** is the one that knows.
**Ofloxacin**, a fluoroquinolone drop,
Stops **bacteria's growth** and makes the pain stop.
Used for **otitis externa**—swimmer's ear fame,
Or **middle ear infections** with a tympanostomy name.
It fights infection right where it starts,
Clearing up pus and painful parts.

It stops the bugs from **copying DNA**,
So bacteria break down and fade away.
**Given by drops**, warm in hand,
Let it settle while they still or stand.
**Side effects?** Just a few to know—
A little **itching**, or a **mild burn flow**.
But reactions are rare and usually pass,
With **relief setting in**, often quite fast.

**Teach caregivers** how to tilt the head,
Pull the ear **back and up** (unless younger instead).

**Five to ten minutes** lying still,

Let the drops soak in, nice and chill.

**Don't touch the tip** to skin or hair,

To keep the bottle clean and fair.

Use the full course—even if clear—

To make sure infection won't reappear.

There's **no black box**, but nurses teach

That antibiotic drops must reach

**Only the ear**, not the eye or mouth,

And keep them stored at room—not south.

Ofloxacin helps when **ear pain strikes**,

For swimmers, kids, and playground hikes.

With **nurse-led care**, and timing wise,

It soothes the ear and quiets cries.

# Omeprazole (Prilosec)

*Proton Pump Inhibitor (PPI)*

When **tummies burn** and **acid flows**,
**Prilosec** helps the healing grow.
**Omeprazole** blocks the pump inside,
Where stomach acid likes to hide.
It shuts down **proton pumps** with might,
So less acid forms—both day and night.
Used for **GERD**, **ulcers**, and **gastritis pain**,
It brings relief to the GI train.

**Given by mouth**, before they eat,
On an **empty stomach** for full defeat.
It comes in **granules**, **tabs**, or **liquid form**,
Just don't crush it—that breaks the norm.
**Side effects?** A few to show:
**Headache**, **nausea**, or a tummy low.
Sometimes **gas**, or a bit of bloat,
But most kids handle it fine by note.

**Long-term use?** Then we stay aware—
Of **low magnesium**, or **fracture care**.

May also **reduce B12** uptake,

So check those labs if symptoms wake.

There's **no black box**, but teach the crew:

It's not a med for every flu.

Used when acid's **chronic and real**,

Not just for one night's fast food meal.

And tell caregivers: **stick to the plan**,

Take it **once daily**, as best they can.

**Don't stop abruptly**, especially in teens—

Rebound acid can be mean.

Omeprazole helps calm the storm,

When bellies burn and pain is the norm.

With **nurse support** and GI insight,

It helps kids sleep through the reflux fight.

# Ondansetron (Zofran)

*Antiemetic; 5-HT3 Receptor Antagonist*

When **nausea hits** and kids feel grim,
**Zofran** helps when the world starts to spin.
**Ondansetron** blocks the gut-brain wire,
That sends **vomiting signals** higher and higher.
Used for **chemo**, **post-op**, or **viral bug**,
It gives little tummies a gentle hug.
It blocks **serotonin's emetic path**,
To settle the stomach and calm the wrath.

**Given by mouth, IV, or ODT tab**,
Dissolves on the tongue—easy grab.
**Every 8 hours**, or as prescribed,
It helps when hydration is hard to revive.
**Side effects?** Usually none,
But sometimes **headache** joins the run.
**Constipation**, **drowsy**, or a bit of a chill,
But most kids tolerate it well and still.

**Caution for QT prolongation**,
Especially with other med combination.

So check that **EKG** if risk is known,

And monitor **electrolytes** that have flown.

There's **no black box**, but **nurse must track**,

Any **rhythm changes** or symptoms back.

Not for **routine stomach bugs** each day—

Use it right, in the proper way.

Teach parents to watch and wait,

And avoid giving more than the dosing rate.

Zofran helps when nothing stays,

To get kids through those queasy days.

With **nurse support**, and timing true,

It helps the smiles return on cue.

# Oseltamivir (Tamiflu)

*Antiviral; Neuraminidase Inhibitor*

When **flu comes fast** with chills and ache,
**Tamiflu** helps the body brake.
**Oseltamivir** works inside,
To stop the virus before it can ride.
It **blocks neuraminidase**, the viral tool,
So flu can't spread and take more rule.
Used for **influenza A and B**,
To shorten symptoms and boost recovery.

Best when started **within two days**,
Of coughs or fevers in flu-filled haze.
Also used for **prophylaxis mode**,
When flu's been shared in the same zip code.
**Given by mouth**, in **capsule or syrup**,
Twice a day, with food as a stir-up.
For five days straight, you finish the course,
Even if symptoms take a gentler course.

**Side effects?** A few to know:
**Nausea**, **vomiting**, or tummy woe.

Some kids feel **dizzy**, others feel off,
And **rare behavior changes** may cause a scoff.
Watch for **hallucinations**, **nightmares**, or fear—
Though rare, these signs mean stay near.
**No black box warning**, but monitor tight,
Especially in kids who don't feel right.

**Not a flu cure**, but a flu fight tool,
That works best with rest, hydration, and rule.
And it won't help with any old cold—
Only the flu, once it's confirmed and bold.
Tamiflu's swift when the flu begins,
To ease the aches and lessen the spins.
With **nurse direction** and time on track,
It helps little bodies start bouncing back.

# Oxcarbazepine (Trileptal)

*Anticonvulsant; Mood Stabilizer*

When **seizures start** and storms arise,
**Trileptal** helps the signals stabilize.
**Oxcarbazepine**, quiet and strong,
Keeps the brain from firing wrong.
It works by **blocking sodium gates**,
To calm the nerve that miscommunicates.
Used for **partial seizures**, young and grown,
And sometimes for **mood** when emotions roam.

It's **by mouth**, in **liquid or tab**,
Twice a day—simple grab.
**Start low and go slow** is the golden plan,
To help the brain adjust as it can.
Side effects? Some kids may feel:
**Drowsiness**, **dizzy**, or off-balance appeal.
**Nausea**, **blurred vision**, or mood that swings,
Even **headaches** or tingling things.

But nurses must **watch sodium drop**,
**Hyponatremia** is a real stop.

Check for **confusion, weakness**, or cramp—
It's not just fatigue or a bedtime lamp.
Rare reactions? They still exist:
Like **rash**, or **Stevens-Johnson twist**.
So educate families what to seek,
And when to call if symptoms peak.

There's **no black box**, but still proceed,
With **labs, mood checks**, and nurse-led speed.
And never stop cold—**taper it slow**,
To keep those seizure risks low.
With **Trileptal**, the brain finds peace,
And daily chaos may start to cease.
With nurse support and proper track,
It helps kids feel more like themselves back.

# Penicillin V (Pen-Vee K)

*Beta-Lactam Antibiotic (Natural Penicillin)*

When **throats are sore** and **germs take hold**,
**Pen-Vee K** fights strong and bold.
**Penicillin V** is tried and true,
A classic med for the bug-fighting crew.
It stops the bacteria from **building walls**,
So the infection weakens, crumbles, and falls.
Great for **strep throat**, **scarlet fever**, and more,
And some **dental infections** doctors deplore.

**Given by mouth**, it's best on time,
Every **6 to 8 hours**—nurse's prime.
Take it **on an empty stomach**, if they can,
Or with food if upset's part of the plan.
**Side effects**? A few may show:
**Nausea**, **diarrhea**, or rash may grow.
And though it's rare, we stay alert,
For **anaphylaxis**, which can hurt.

Ask about allergies—very key!
Especially to **penicillin family**.

If signs of **wheezing**, **rash**, or **shock**,
Stop the dose and call the doc.
No **black box warning**, but teach with care,
To **finish the course**, even if they swear
They're "feeling fine"—it's not a reason
To stop too early mid-antibiotic season.

Store **liquid form** in the fridge just right,
And **shake it well** before each night.
Measure it out with a proper tool,
No kitchen spoons in nursing school!
Pen-Vee K is simple and strong,
With decades of use—it's rarely wrong.
With **nurse guidance** and parent trust,
It clears the bugs and does what it must.

# Permethrin (Elimite, Nix)

*Topical Scabicide & Pediculicide*

When **itchy bugs** won't go away,
**Permethrin** helps to save the day.
**Elimite** for **scabies**, **Nix** for **lice**,
This medicated cream feels nice (and precise).
It **paralyzes pests** in skin and hair,
So mites and lice don't stand a prayer.
It's used in kids for those tiny foes,
From **burrowing bugs** to **nit-lined rows**.

For **scabies**, rub it **neck to toes**,
Leave it on while the little one dozes.
Wash it off in **8 to 14 hours**,
Then clean the clothes, the sheets, the towers.
For **lice**, use **shampoo-style Nix**,
Leave it on for **10 minutes**—quick fix!
Then rinse it out and **comb the strands**,
To remove the eggs with careful hands.

**Side effects?** Mostly **mild and brief**—
**Redness**, **itching**, or skin relief.

Some may feel a slight **tingle or burn**,
But that just means it's taking its turn.
Teach families: one dose may not be all,
A **repeat in 7 days** might be the call.
Clean **brushes**, **bedding**, and things that touch hair,
So lice don't hide and reappear there.

There's **no black box**, but education's key—
To prevent **reinfection** in the family tree.
Don't use it near **eyes**, or on **open skin**,
And ask before use if **younger than two in**.
Permethrin stops the itch and squirm,
In **lice that crawl** and **mites that worm**.
With **nurse direction** and parent might,
It clears the bugs and sleeps the night.

# Phenobarbital

*Barbiturate Anticonvulsant; Sedative-Hypnotic*

When **seizures strike** in babies small,
**Phenobarbital** helps calm it all.
A **barbiturate**, old but true,
It slows the brain like few meds do.
It enhances **GABA's calming gate**,
To slow down signals that miscommunicate.
Used for **neonatal seizures**, **epilepsy**, too,
And sometimes as a **sedative** for breakthrough.

**Given IV, IM, or oral in drops**,
It works for hours before it stops.
But it builds up in tissues deep—
So nurses watch for **sedative sleep**.
**Side effects?** A sleepy haze,
With **lethargy** that can last for days.
**Ataxia, hyperactivity,** or **rash**,
And **cognitive delays** if used in a flash.

Long-term use can **slow down growth**,
So weigh the risks before you oath.

It may cause **tolerance**, even **dependence**,
So tapering plans require attendance.
**Black box warning?** Yes, it's there—
For **addiction, abuse,** and **breathing care.**
**Respiratory depression** may arise,
So **monitor closely**—no compromise.

Check **drug levels**, labs, and signs,
Track **liver, CBC,** and **enzyme lines.**
And don't stop cold—**withdrawal's rough,**
With **seizures, irritability,** and all that stuff.
Teach families to **dose with care,**
And **keep it locked**, not anywhere.
Though old-school, it still holds a place,
When newer meds can't match the pace.

With **nurse support**, and close review,
Phenobarb helps when nothing else will do.
A steady hand, a quiet tide—
To help young minds grow safe inside.

# Phenylephrine (Sudafed PE)

*Decongestant; Alpha-1 Adrenergic Agonist*

When **tiny noses** get stuffy and tight,
**Sudafed PE** can bring back the light.
**Phenylephrine** works to shrink the swell,
Inside the nose where congestion dwells.
It's an **alpha-1 agonist**, smooth and neat,
That **clamps down vessels** so kids can breathe sweet.
Used for **cold**, **sinus**, and **allergy days**,
It clears up passages clouded in haze.

**Given by mouth** in syrup or tab,
But not for infants—and that's no fab.
**Under four years?** It's not advised,
Due to **side effects** often disguised.
**Side effects** may start to show:
**Irritability**, **headache**, or a **heart that goes go**.
Sometimes **sleeplessness** joins the ride,
Or **increased BP** lurking inside.

**Short-term use** is what we teach,
Just a **few days**—then stop the reach.

Too much can cause **rebound stuff**,
Where congestion returns even rough.
No **black box warning**, but caution true,
Especially in **kids with heart issues** too.
Avoid with other **stimulant meds**,
And teach parents all that nursing says.

And here's the kicker: it's **less effective**
Than **pseudoephedrine**, though still elective.
But since it's OTC and found in blends,
It's often picked by well-meaning friends.
So **nurses guide** with careful voice,
Helping families make a safer choice.
Phenylephrine works in a pinch or two,
With short-term relief and nursing view.

# Pimecrolimus Cream (Elidel)

*Topical Calcineurin Inhibitor; Non-Steroidal Anti-Inflammatory*

When **eczema flares** and skin turns red,
But **steroid creams** aren't where you're led,
**Elidel** steps in, calm and thin,
To help the healing gently begin.
**Pimecrolimus** is the name it owns,
It **blocks T-cells** and **inflammatory zones**.
It calms the skin's immune alarm,
Without the **thinning steroid charm**.

Used for **mild to moderate eczema pain**,
Especially on **face**, where steroids strain.
Apply it **twice daily**—thin and neat,
Until the rash begins retreat.
It's for kids **two and older** in age,
And always used with a **moisture gauge**.
**No occlusive dressings**, let it breathe,
And **wash your hands** each time you leave.

**Side effects?** Some feel a **burn or sting**,

Especially when eczema's in full swing.
Rarely **redness**, **itch**, or local heat,
But those pass by as skin repeats.
There **is a black box warning**, be aware:
For a **theoretical cancer scare**.
Though no strong link has yet been shown,
Families deserve the risks well-known.

Teach parents to use it just as told,
And not for **infections**, **fungus**, or **cold**.
If skin gets worse or oozes pus,
They should stop and follow up with us.
Elidel gives the skin a chance
To breathe and heal without the dance
Of steroid risks when used too long—
With **nursing care**, the choice is strong.

# Pneumococcal Vaccine (Prevnar 13)

*Conjugate Vaccine (PCV13) – Streptococcus pneumoniae Protection*

When **pneumonia looms** or **earaches strike**,

**Prevnar 13** guards kids alike.

A **pneumococcal vaccine** strong and smart,

It teaches the body how to play its part.

It protects from **thirteen bacterial strains**,

That cause **meningitis**, **lungs**, and **ear pains**.

It stops infections from getting deep,

And helps little ones eat, play, and sleep.

**Given IM** in a little thigh,

At **2, 4, 6 months**, then a **booster at five**.

It builds up shields from very young,

So serious illness won't be among.

Side effects? They're **mild and brief**—

Like a **sore arm**, or a touch of grief.

Maybe a **fever**, or **fussiness** flare,

But nothing beyond good nursing care.

**No black box warning**, but teach the why—

**Strep pneumo** infections can terrify.

They can spread through **blood**, **lungs**, or **brain**,

Causing **sepsis**, **deafness**, or lasting pain.

Teach caregivers this one's key,

To protect from bugs they'll never see.

And if a child is **immune weak**,

This vaccine becomes even more unique.

Prevnar builds **community walls**,

To stop big bugs from making calls.

With **nurse guidance** and a sticker prize,

It helps our babies immunize.

# Polyethylene Glycol (MiraLAX)
*Osmotic Laxative*

When **bowels slow down** and stools get tight,
**MiraLAX** helps things move just right.
**Polyethylene glycol**, powder and plain,
Brings **water to stool** to ease the strain.
It's **tasteless**, mixed with juice or tea,
So kids will drink it willingly.
Used for **occasional or chronic** delay,
It helps kids poop without dismay.

It **draws in water** to soften the load,
So stool moves gently down the road.
It's **not a stimulant**, no harsh surprise,
Just steady work without the cries.
**Given by mouth**, once daily is best,
But **dosing by weight** helps avoid the mess.
Start low and adjust as needed true—
And don't forget **hydration**, too!

**Side effects** are mild and rare:
**Gas**, **cramps**, or a looser affair.

But no electrolyte shifts in sight,
Which makes it safer day and night.
**No black box warning**, but teach the way—
This isn't forever, just day by day.
Pair it with **fiber**, fruits, and play,
So bowels learn to go their way.

Teach families to **mix it well**,
And **don't expect magic right when it's dealt**.
It may take a **day or two** to act,
But when it does, it's smooth and packed.
MiraLAX gives relief with grace,
No battles, tears, or bathroom chase.
With **nurse support** and dosing clear,
It brings those bowels back into gear.

# Prednisolone (Orapred, Prelone)

*Corticosteroid; Anti-Inflammatory*

When **inflammation flares** or **airways swell**,
**Orapred** helps the body do well.
**Prednisolone**, a steroid strong,
Tells the immune system, "Not for long!"
Used for **asthma**, **allergies**, **croupy cough**,
Or rashes that just won't back off.
Also helps when joints inflame,
Or autoimmune flares call out a name.

It works by **suppressing cytokine flow**,
To calm down cells that start the show.
Given **by mouth**, as **liquid or tab**,
Once or twice daily, based on the lab.
**Short-term use** brings power fast,
But **long-term use** can be a blast...
Of **mood swings**, **weight gain**, **tummy woes**,
And **blood sugar spikes**—as the steroid grows.

Side effects include:
 **Irritability**,

**Insomnia,**

**Increased appetite**—instantly!

And don't forget **GI distress**,

So give it **with food** to limit the mess.

**Tapering's needed** if used long-term,

To let the adrenal glands reconfirm.

Stopping cold can cause a crash,

So nurses teach to **ease, not dash**.

There's **no black box**, but watch the signs—

Of **infection masked**, or **emotional lines**.

It lowers defense while calming the flame,

So teach families it's not a game.

Prednisolone soothes what's inflamed inside,

Helping kids breathe, move, or rest with pride.

With **nurse support**, timed just right,

It brings the body back to light.

# Prednisolone Acetate Ophthalmic (Pred Forte)

*Ophthalmic Corticosteroid (Anti-Inflammatory Eye Drop)*

When **eyes are red** and swollen tight,
**Pred Forte** helps restore the light.
**Prednisolone acetate**, in drop form so clear,
Calms the eye when pain draws near.
Used for **uveitis, injuries**, and post-surgical care,
Or **allergic inflammation** lingering there.
It eases the itch, the haze, the burn,
And helps those tired eyes return.

It's a **steroid drop**, not for the nose,
And not for infections that secretly grow.
If **viral or fungal** bugs are to blame,
Steroid drops can worsen the game.
**Shake well** before you give each dose,
Because suspensions settle more than most.
**1 to 2 drops**, as ordered in line,
Every few hours or spaced by time.

**Side effects** may include:

**Blurred vision**,

**Pressure that's rude**,

So monitor for **IOP rise**,

Especially in kids with glaucoma eyes.

**Stinging**, **burning**, or **drying too**,

But usually short and nothing new.

Use **clean hands**, and don't touch the tip—

Contamination is a slippery trip.

There's **no black box**, but we still teach:

To use it only where **orders reach**.

And **don't stop suddenly** without the say,

As rebound inflammation can find its way.

Pred Forte's strong, but best when led

By **nurse direction** and what the provider said.

It calms the fire behind the stare,

Bringing comfort, sight, and healing care.

# Prednisone

*Systemic Corticosteroid; Anti-Inflammatory; Immunosuppressant*

When **inflammation rages** deep inside,

**Prednisone** helps turn the tide.

From **asthma flares** to **autoimmune pain**,

It tells the immune system to **restrain**.

It **mimics cortisol**, strong and bold,

To **reduce swelling**, **heat**, and hold.

Used for **allergies, arthritis, Crohn's**, and more,

Even **croup** or **nephrotic** cases we store.

**Given by mouth**, in **tablet or syrup**,

It's often **once daily** in a morning setup.

**Short bursts** for a flare? It acts fast and clean—

But **long-term use** can turn unseen.

Side effects? Let's list the crew:

**Mood swings**,

**Hunger**,

**Tummy flu**,

**Insomnia, acne**, or a **rounder face**,

Even **slowed growth** in a chronic case.

It may **raise blood sugar**, **lower bone**,

And **suppress immunity** all on its own.

So nurses teach and families track,

All changes small or symptoms back.

Never stop **cold**—that's a rule we hold,

Or the **adrenals** crash and symptoms unfold.

Taper it **slowly** if the course is long,

With nurse-led care to guide what's strong.

No **black box**, but still a star,

In managing flares that go too far.

Teach to take it **with food**, not plain,

To guard the stomach from steroid strain.

Prednisone's power is best when planned,

With **timed doses**, a **steady hand**.

It calms the body when storms ignite—

With **nursing support**, it sets things right.

# Promethazine (Phenergan)

*Antihistamine (First-Generation); Antiemetic; Sedative*

When **nausea strikes** or **motion sways**,
**Phenergan** helps in tricky days.
**Promethazine**, old-school and strong,
Can ease a tummy that's felt wrong too long.
It blocks **H1 histamine** at the gate,
And calms the brain's emetic state.
Used for **vomiting, allergies,** or **pre-op ease**,
And sometimes for a **sedating breeze**.

**Given by mouth, IM,** or **rectal, too,**
But **never IV push**—that's a safety cue.
For kids, it must be used with care—
Too much can lead to real despair.
**Black box warning** in bold and loud:
**Respiratory depression** in the younger crowd.
**Under age two**, it's not approved,
And **older kids** must be carefully moved.

**Side effects?** They often include:
**Sedation,**

**Dizziness,**

**Shifts in mood.**

Also **dry mouth, blurred sight**, and more,

So monitor closely and explore.

It may cause **extrapyramidal signs**,

Like **dystonia, twitches**, or **rigid lines**.

And rarely, **neuroleptic syndrome** appears,

So we educate families to spot the fears.

Teach parents it's not for every upset,

Not for **routine nausea** or cold's onset.

And **don't combine** with sedatives near,

To avoid a mix that's unsafe here.

Promethazine works when used with grace,

In **older children**, the **right time and place**.

With **nurse guidance**, dose, and care,

It soothes the system and clears the air.

# Pseudoephedrine (Sudafed)

*Decongestant; Alpha/Beta Adrenergic Agonist*

When **sinuses swell** and breathing's tight,
**Sudafed** helps the airflow right.
**Pseudoephedrine** shrinks the space,
Where mucus clogs and floods the place.
It's an **alpha agonist**, strong and quick,
That **constricts the vessels** to clear up thick.
Used for **nasal stuffiness**, **sinus pain**,
It helps dry out the congestion train.

**Given by mouth**, it lasts a while,
But **watch the dose** and keep it mild.
It's **not for kids under age four**,
And even in older ones—**use no more than before**.

**Side effects?** They're energy-fueled:
**Nervousness**,
**Fast heart**,
**Tempers unruled**.
Also **headache**, **tummy upset**, or **can't sleep**,
So give it **early**, not in the nighttime sweep.

This med is **controlled** in many a state,
Because of **meth use** it can create.
So it's behind-the-counter—no grab and go,
And **caregiver education** is key to know.
**No black box warning**, but safety's tight,
Especially with **heart** or **thyroid** fight.
Avoid in kids with **hypertension**,
And **don't combine** without full attention.

Teach to **read labels**, and never stack,
Cold meds often **double it back**.
So Sudafed use should be brief and wise,
Just a few days before symptoms disguise.
Pseudoephedrine clears the head,
But needs a **nurse and parent** lead instead.
With short-term plans and mindful track,
It helps the breathing pathways crack.

# Risperidone (Risperdal)

*Atypical Antipsychotic; Mood Stabilizer*

When **thoughts run wild** or **rage runs deep**,
**Risperdal** helps the brain find sleep.
**Risperidone**, calm and slow,
Helps **mood** and **behavior** gently flow.
Used for **autism-related aggression**,
**Irritability**, or **psychotic depression**.
Also for **bipolar** and **schizophrenic strain**,
To soften delusions or racing brain.

It **blocks dopamine and serotonin gates**,
To regulate mood and stabilize states.
**Given by mouth**, as **liquid or tab**,
Dosed by weight with a careful grab.

**Side effects** may come in waves:
**Drowsiness**,
**Dizziness**,
**Big appetite craves**.
**Weight gain** and **hormonal rise**,
(Like **gynecomastia** in some young guys).

Watch for **tremors**, **stiffness**, or a **frozen gait**,
Signs of **EPS**—don't hesitate.
And **tardive dyskinesia**, though rare, is real—
So nurses assess how the child feels.

There's a **black box warning** (nurses know),
For **elderly use**, where **stroke risks grow**.
But still, we teach with extra care,
Because side effects can surface anywhere.
**Labs to monitor**: weight, glucose, lipids, too—
And mental health checks as kids push through.
Start **low and slow**, then build if right,
And track for signs both day and night.

Risperidone can **ground the storm**,
When used with care, it can transform.
With **nursing support**, a team in sync,
It helps young minds come back from the brink.

# Senna (Senokot)
*Stimulant Laxative*

When **tummies are stuck** and bowels won't go,
**Senokot** helps to start the flow.
**Senna** is nature's push and prod,
To help the colon do its job.
It **stimulates muscles** in the gut,
So stool can move and kids aren't stuck.
Used for **constipation**, short and slow,
It helps those hard-to-pass stools go.

It's **by mouth**, in **syrup**, **tablet**, or **tea**,
And often works in **6 to 12 hours**, you'll see.
Best when taken **right before bed**,
So morning relief lies just ahead.
**Side effects?** You may spot:
**Cramping**,
**Diarrhea**,
**Loose or hot**.
**Electrolyte loss** with chronic use,
So don't let it become a daily excuse.

**No black box warning**, but still proceed
With **hydration**, fiber, and dosing heed.
Teach caregivers it's **not forever**,
Just a **gentle nudge**, not a full-time lever.
It may turn **stools yellow, red, or brown**,
And that's okay—don't write it down.
But if kids still struggle more than a few,
A provider should take a closer view.

Senna helps when things slow low,
But **nurse support** helps rhythm grow.
With timing, balance, and routine smart,
Senokot plays a helpful part.

# Sertraline (Zoloft)

*Selective Serotonin Reuptake Inhibitor (SSRI); Antidepressant*

When **feelings are heavy** or **worries don't slow**,

**Zoloft** helps the healing grow.

**Sertraline** lifts the fog and fear,

So kids can feel more present here.

It blocks the **reuptake of serotonin's light**,

So more can flow and moods feel right.

Used for **depression**, **OCD**, and **anxious minds**,

It helps calm thoughts of all kinds.

**Given by mouth**, once a day,

Usually in the **morning** to clear the way.

**Start low and go slow** is key,

As side effects can temporarily be.

They may feel:

**Nausea**,

**Vivid dreams**,

**Sleepy** or **wired**—it swings between.

Sometimes **appetite** shifts or a **headache**, too,

But many resolve once levels are through.

**Black box warning**—loud and clear:

For **suicidal thoughts** in youth, we steer.

So nurses and parents must **closely track**,

Behavioral shifts and mood that's off track.

Not to be **stopped cold**—that's rough,

**Taper slowly** if they've had enough.

Watch for **serotonin syndrome** signs,

Like **sweating**, **confusion**, or **twitchy lines**.

**Teach caregivers** what to expect,

That healing's slow and not direct.

It may take **weeks** to feel the lift,

But Zoloft can be a steady gift.

With **nurse support** and mental health care,

Sertraline helps kids rise from despair.

It's not a cure, but a stable floor,

To help them feel themselves once more.

# Silver Sulfadiazine Cream (Silvadene)

*Topical Antibacterial; Sulfa-Based Burn Cream*

When **burns are raw** and skin's in pain,
**Silvadene** helps to soothe the flame.
**Silver sulfadiazine**, cool and white,
Fights off bugs and brings down fright.
It's used for **partial-** and **full-thickness burns**,
To stop infection before it returns.
The **silver kills bacteria** on the skin,
While **sulfa** helps keep healing in.

Apply it **topically**, clean and thin,
With sterile gloves on—never just skin.
Usually done **once or twice a day**,
Or with dressings changed the wound-care way.
**Side effects?** Not often, but still:
A **burning**, **itching**, or **rash-like chill**.
Sometimes **leukopenia** shows on the sheet,
So nurses track the **CBC beat**.

Don't use it in kids with **sulfa allergies**,

Or on **face**, **near eyes**, or **mucosal territories**.

And **not for newborns** in the first few days—

It raises **bilirubin** in risky ways.

No **black box warning**, but teach the rule:

It's **for burns**, not a general wound-care tool.

And if the skin turns **gray or blue**,

That's **silver staining** coming through.


Silvadene cools when burns feel hot,

And helps infections find their spot.

With **nurse-led care** and sterile touch,

It protects the skin without too much.

# Simethicone (Mylicon)

*Anti-Gas Agent; Antifoaming Agent*

When **baby tummies** rumble with air,
**Mylicon** helps bring comfort there.
**Simethicone** breaks up the foam,
So gas can pass and peace comes home.
It works by **reducing surface tension**,
Letting bubbles burst without much mention.
Used for **colic**, **gassy cries**, or **post-feed swell**,
It helps little ones feel more well.

**Given by mouth**, in **drops or chew**,
**After meals** or at **bedtime**, too.
It's **not absorbed**, just works on gut—
So it's safe, even in newborns' rut.
**Side effects?** Hardly a trace—
It's gentle, calm, and leaves no race.
No sedation, no stomach woe,
Just easier gas to let it go.

No **black box warning**, and no alarms,
Just teach to **dose with gentle arms**.

**Clean the dropper, shake it well,**

And **pair with burping**—that helps as well.

Teach parents it's a **supportive friend**,

Not a cure, but a means to an end.

With warm hands, timing, and nursing grace,

Simethicone makes room in that tiny space.

# Sodium Chloride 0.9% IV

When **volume drops** or veins run dry,
**Normal Saline** comes standing by.
**Sodium chloride**, at **point-nine percent**,
Is the fluid most commonly sent.
It's **isotonic**, matching blood's tone,
So cells stay stable, not overblown.
Used for **dehydration**, **shock**, or **flush**,
Or to **dilute meds** in a careful rush.

Given **IV**, in bags or syringes,
It flows through lines and tubing hinges.
Whether **bolus** or **maintenance drip**,
It keeps perfusion firm in grip.

**Side effects?** They're rarely seen,
But too much fluid's not so clean.
Watch for signs of **fluid overload**—
**Edema**, **crackles**, or **respiratory load**.

No **black box warning**, but nurses assess

**Electrolytes**, **output**, and fluid stress.
And if it's running in a fragile vein,
Monitor closely to avoid pain.
It contains just **salt and water**, plain,
But in the body, it holds great gain.
Used in trauma, fever, or thirst,
It's often the first line we disperse.

Teach parents not to confuse the kind—
It's **not the same** as saline for behind!
This one's **for veins**, not wounds or nose,
It's IV therapy that gently flows.
Sodium chloride, a steady stream,
Supports the heart and every team.
With **nurse-led checks** and fluid cues,
It helps small patients safely cruise.

# Sulfamethoxazole/Trimethoprim (Bactrim, Septra)

When **fevers rise** and **bugs resist**,
**Bactrim** steps in with a double twist.
**Sulfamethoxazole** and **Trimethoprim** blend,
To stop bacteria end-to-end.
They block two steps in **folate's track**,
So bugs can't grow or double back.
Used for **UTIs**, **MRSA**, **ear**, and **gut**,
And **pneumocystis** when immune's in a rut.

**Given by mouth**, or sometimes **IV**,
With **weight-based dosing** carefully.
Take it with **water** to guard the kidney,
And **after meals** to calm the tummy.

Side effects? A list to scan:
**Fever**,
**Rash**,
**GI cramp plan**.
Sometimes **photosensitivity**,

So **limit sun**—that's nurse activity.

Also watch for **Stevens-Johnson's rare**,

A **severe skin reaction** needing urgent care.

Check **CBCs** and **renal labs**,

Especially in kids with health that drabs.

It's **not for infants under two months**,

Or kids with **sulfa allergy fronts**.

And not with **warfarin**—it boosts effect,

So review med lists and double-check.

**No black box warning**, but we still teach,

That **hydration** is within nurse reach.

And **complete the full course**, no matter what,

Even when symptoms feel forgot.

Bactrim's strong with a double swing,

Fighting bugs with a one-two zing.

With **nurse-led care** and timing neat,

It helps infections face defeat.

# Tacrolimus Ointment (Protopic)

*Topical Calcineurin Inhibitor; Non-Steroidal Anti-Inflammatory*

When **eczema flares** and steroids aren't right,
**Protopic** steps in to calm the fight.
**Tacrolimus** ointment, smooth and clear,
Soothes the skin without thinning fear.
It blocks **T-cell signals** in the skin,
To stop the itch before it begins.
Used for **moderate to severe atopic plight**,
Especially on the **face**, where skin is light.

Apply it **thin, twice a day**,
To affected spots—not a spray-and-pray.
**No occlusion**, and **clean, dry skin**,
Let it absorb before clothes go in.

**Side effects?** Some kids may feel:
**Stinging**,
**Burning**,
A **warm-faced deal**.
Often fades as skin adapts,

But keep track if the reaction lasts.

**Black box warning**, bold and bright:
For a **possible cancer risk** in sight.
Though no strong link is firmly shown,
It's best to use when alternatives are blown.
Not for **infants under two**,
And not for **fungal, viral,** or **bacterial** too.
It's not for daily use all year—
Just **flares**, short-term, when rash draws near.

Teach families to **wash hands after**,
And avoid the eyes—that's nursing chatter.
**No sun or tanning** while this is on,
As **UV risk** is slightly drawn.
Protopic calms with a **steroid-free grace**,
For delicate skin on the **neck and face**.
With **nurse support**, it finds its place,
In healing flares without a trace.

# Tobramycin

*Aminoglycoside Antibiotic (Ophthalmic Use)*

When **eyes are red** and filled with goop,
**Tobrex** helps clear up the soup.
**Tobramycin**, an antibiotic drop,
Stops **bacterial growth** and makes it stop.
It blocks the bugs' **protein plan**,
So they can't spread or make a stand.
Used for **conjunctivitis**, gritty or sore,
Or other **eye infections** that knock on the door.

**Given by drops** or **ointment form**,
It works through days both calm and storm.
**One to two drops, every four to six**,
Or as prescribed—just don't self-mix.
**Side effects?** They're usually mild:
A **burning, stinging**, or a **watery child**.
But if there's **rash, itch**, or swelling seen,
Stop and call—it could mean something mean.

Not for **viral** or **fungal** eye invasion,
This one's for **bacterial inflammation**.

And don't share bottles—cross-contamination's real,

Teach caregivers that part of the deal.

**No black box warning**, but we advise,

Use **as ordered**—not just when eyes surprise.

Wash hands well before each dose,

And **don't touch the tip**—that's gross and close.

Finish the course, even if clear,

To stop the bugs from reappearing near.

Tobrex helps when eyes revolt,

With **nursing care**, it halts the jolt.

# Topical Lidocaine/Prilocaine (EMLA Cream)

*Topical Anesthetic Combination*

When **shots bring fear** or **IVs sting**,
**EMLA cream** helps soften the thing.
**Lidocaine and prilocaine** paired just right,
To numb the skin and ease the fright.
It blocks the nerves in the upper skin,
So pain can't travel deep within.
Used before **needles**, **lines**, or **cuts**,
It calms the flinch and quiets the guts.

Apply it **thick**, then **cover tight**,
With **occlusive dressing** sealed just right.
Wait **at least 30 to 60 minutes**, true,
For full effect to follow through.

**Side effects?** A few may feel:
A **redness**, **blanching**, or **tingling peel**.
Rarely **paleness** or a **mild rash**,
But reactions fade away in a flash.

Don't use on **broken skin** or **open sore**,
Or in **infants under 3 months** (or more).
Too much can cause **methemoglobinemia**,
Which turns the blood blue in a scary schema.

**No black box warning**, but still go slow—
And teach parents what they need to know.
**Dose by weight**, and limit the space,
To avoid systemic numbing in any case.
**Don't rub it in**, and wash off clean,
Before the procedure steps on the scene.
And always label the site that's done—
To prevent confusion from patient to one.

EMLA brings **comfort before the poke**,
So fewer tears and less kiddo choke.
With **nurse timing**, trust, and care,
Even scary stuff feels fair.

# Triamcinolone Cream (Kenalog)

*Topical Corticosteroid (Medium Potency)*

When **rashes itch** or **eczema flares**,
**Kenalog** helps with skin repair.
**Triamcinolone**, smooth and strong,
Calms inflammation that's gone on too long.
It lowers **swelling**, **itch**, and **red**,
Where allergic skin reactions spread.
Used for **dermatitis**, **bug bites**, too,
And **psoriasis plaques** in a stubborn hue.

**Apply a thin layer**, **once or twice** a day,
Only on skin that the doc says, "Okay."
No **face**, **groin**, or **diaper zone**,
Unless prescribed for those spots alone.
**Side effects?** They're mostly light:
A little **burning**, **stinging**, or **skin too tight**.
But **long-term use** can cause some strife—
Like **thinning skin** or **color life**.

No **black box warning**, but here's our stance:
**Don't use it like lotion**—no daily dance.

It's for flares, not for a forever fix,
And not to be mixed with home-remedy tricks.
Teach caregivers to **wash hands before**,
Apply the cream, then **wash once more**.
Don't cover with bandage unless told to do,
That can **trap the med** and cause more too.

Triamcinolone calms the storm,
When skin is red and far from norm.
With **nurse advice** and a healing tone,
Kenalog helps bring comfort home.

# Trimethoprim/Sulfamethoxazole (Bactrim)

*Combination Antibiotic; Sulfonamide Class*

When **bacteria dig in** and won't let go,
**Bactrim** helps put on a show.
It's **trimethoprim** and **sulfa**, paired just right,
To block the bugs from gaining might.
They **stop folic acid** in two-step ways,
So bacteria stall in their growing phase.
Used for **UTIs**, **MRSA**, **ear**, and **gut**,
And **pneumocystis** when immunity's cut.

**Given by mouth**, or **IV drip**,
With **weight-based dosing**—nurses don't skip.
Take it with **water**, don't let it stick,
And **don't skip doses**—that's the trick.

**Side effects?** Yep, here's the list:
**Fever**,
**GI twist**,
**Photosensitivity**, sunburn fast,

**Rash** and **labs** that may not last.
But here's the one we always flag:
 **Stevens-Johnson** is a rare red flag.
If **blisters**, **fever**, or **peeling skin** show,
Stop the med and let the provider know.

Not for **babies under two months old**,
And never with **sulfa allergies** bold.
**Drug interactions?** Keep an eye—
**Warfarin**, **phenytoin**, may amplify.
No **black box warning**, but teach with care,
Hydration helps, and so does air.
And **finish the course**, don't stop mid-run,
Even if symptoms seem all done.

Bactrim's bold, with a combo swing,
A one-two punch to zap the thing.
With **nurse guidance** and steady view,
It clears the bugs and pulls kids through.

# Valacyclovir (Valtrex)

*Antiviral; Nucleoside Analog*

When **viruses linger** and cause a sting,
**Valtrex** steps in to clip their wing.
**Valacyclovir**, smooth and clean,
Fights **herpes**, **shingles**, and **cold sore** scenes.
It's a **prodrug** that turns into **acyclovir**,
Which stops the virus from multiplying near.
Used for **HSV-1**, **HSV-2**,
And **chickenpox** if it's early too.

Given **by mouth**, once or twice,
With **weight-based dosing** to keep things nice.
Start it **early**—within the day,
To shorten symptoms and keep pain at bay.
**Side effects?** They're usually tame:
**Nausea**, **headache**, or **tummy game**.
Rarely **dizzy**, or **rash appears**,
But serious reactions are few through the years.

**Hydration is key**—that's a must,
To protect the **kidneys** and gain our trust.

Especially in kids who don't drink well,
**Push fluids** while they're under its spell.
No **black box warning**, but still review,
It's not a cure—but it helps get through.
And though the **virus still can spread**,
It lowers the risk when dosing's led.

Teach families: take it **just as planned**,
And wash those hands when lesions land.
No sharing drinks or towels near—
Until the sores completely clear.
Valacyclovir helps take the edge
Off viral flares from nerve-end wedge.
With **nurse-led care** and dosing tight,
It brings relief and helps kids fight.

# Varicella Vaccine (Varivax)

*Live Attenuated Vaccine – Chickenpox Prevention*

When **itchy spots** begin to spread,
And **fever** dances on a little head,
**Varivax** stops it before it starts—
Protecting skin and little hearts.
It's the **chickenpox vaccine**, given with care,
To keep those **blisters** from popping everywhere.
A **live attenuated** viral shot,
That teaches the body what not to rot.

Given **subcutaneously**, neat and small,
At **12–15 months**, then again before school hall.
The second dose comes at **age four to six**,
To make sure the immunity sticks.
It prevents **itch**, **scars**, and **days in bed**,
And rare but serious risks instead—
Like **pneumonia**, **brain inflammation**, too,
Or **superinfection** sneaking through.

**Side effects?** Just light, don't stress—
A **mild rash**, or **soreness** at the press.

Maybe a **fever**, or feel a bit off,

But rarely more than a brief, light cough.

Teach that it's **live**, so don't give to:

**Immunocompromised**,

**Pregnant**, too.

And **no aspirin** after this vaccine day—

It may raise **Reye's syndrome** risk your way.

**No black box warning**, but nurses teach,

That **two doses** bring strong disease outreach.

And if there's a rash in the days that come,

Avoid newborns until it's done.

Varivax guards with a simple poke,

So kids can laugh, not itch and soak.

With **nurse support** and timing right,

It keeps the chickenpox out of sight.

# Vitamin D3 (Cholecalciferol)

*Vitamin Supplement; Fat-Soluble Nutrient*

When **bones need strength** and **moods feel low**,
**Vitamin D3** helps kids grow.
**Cholecalciferol**, sunshine's friend,
Supports the body from end to end.
It helps absorb **calcium** true,
To build up **teeth** and **skeletons, too**.
It boosts the **immune system**, helps kids fight,
And keeps their muscles working right.

Used for **rickets, low D**, or support each day,
Especially when sun can't find its way.
**Given by mouth**, in **drops or chew**,
Or **capsules** for older children too.
**Infants** need it from early on,
Especially if breast milk is what they're on.
**400 IU** is the daily goal,
To help their little bodies roll.

**Side effects?** Not when it's right—
But too much D can cause a fright:

**Nausea,**

**Thirst,**

**Calcium too high,**

So dosing must be nurse-guided and shy.

**No black box warning**, but don't just guess,
Too much can lead to **calcified mess**.
So teach to follow what docs advise,
And not grab extras in super-size.
Pair it with food that helps it stick—
Like **fatty fish**, or **milk** real quick.
And always track the dosing tool,
Not household spoons—that breaks the rule.

Vitamin D3 fuels kids bright,
With **nurse support** and dosage right.
From **stronger bones** to **smiles that shine**,
This sunshine vitamin helps align.

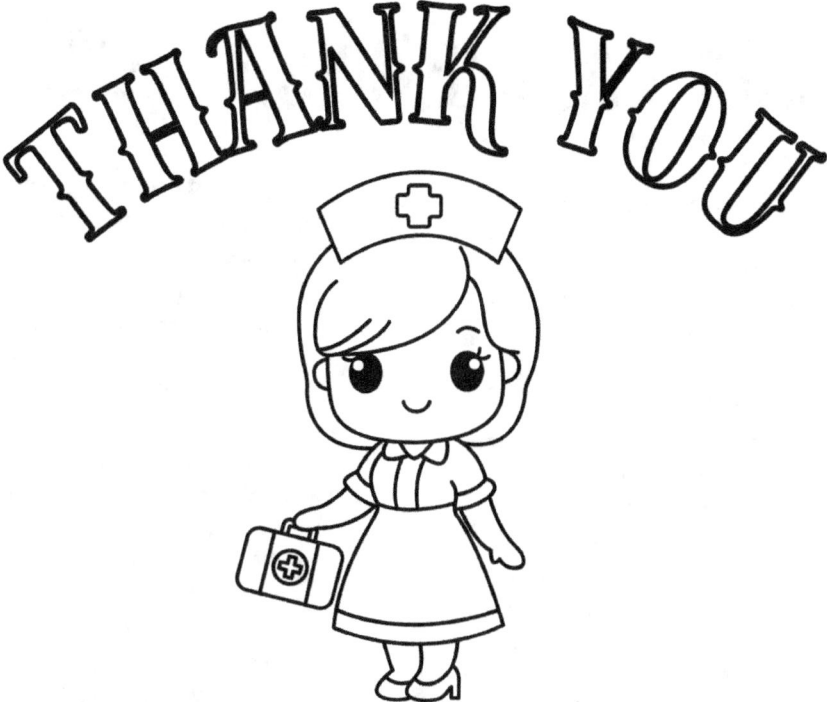

**for getting this book and for making it all the way to the end!**

Before you go, I wanted to ask you for one small favor. Could you please consider posting a review? Because posting a review is the best and easiest way to support the work of independent authors like me.

Your feedback will help me a ton!

Click **Here** or Scan the QR code below!

# OTHER TITLES IN THE MADE EASY SERIES

Geriatrics Made Easy
Emergency Care Made Easy
Critical Care Made Easy
Human Growth & Development
Maternal & Newborn Made Easy
Mental Health Made Easy
Organic Chemistry Made Easy
General Chemistry Made Easy
Pediatrics Made Easy
Med-Surg Made Easy, Vol 1
Med-Surg Made Easy, Vol 2
Microbiology Made Easy
Nursing Skills & Procedures
Pathophysiology Made Easy
Nursing Assessment Made Easy
Nutrition Made Easy
Anatomy & Physiology Vol 1
Anatomy & Physiology Vol 2

### Pharmacology Series
Pharmacology Made Easy Vol 1
Pharmacology Made Easy Vol 2
Pharmacology Made Easy Vol 3
Oncology Meds Made Easy
Cardiac Meds Made Easy
Endocrine Meds Made Easy
Pain Meds Made Easy
GI Meds Made Easy
Respiratory Meds Made Easy
Critical Meds Made Easy
ER/ICU Meds Made Easy
Neuro Meds Made Easy
Psych Meds Made Easy
Pediatric Meds Made Easy
OB/GYN Meds Made Easy

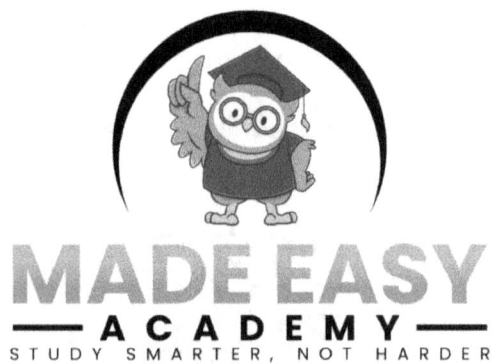